Synopsis of Key Gynecologic Oncology Trials

This revised and updated new edition of a best-selling text remains a fast and convenient overview of the clinical trials in gynecologic cancer treatment, outlining the evidence base of treatment decisions in uterine, ovarian, cervical, and vulvar cancers, and gestational trophoblastic neoplasia. Residents and fellows will find this book an indispensable reference, while practitioners will welcome it as a clarification of the evidence base for treatment options.

- Gives a convenient summary of trials in gynecologic oncology
- Supplies an invaluable revision primer for those undertaking certification
- Provides a uniquely up-to-date resource

Synopsis of Key Gynecologic Oncology Trials

Second Edition

Malte Renz, MD, PhD
Division of Gynecologic Oncology, Stanford University
School of Medicine, Stanford, California, USA

Elisabeth J. Diver, MD
Division of Gynecologic Oncology, Stanford University
School of Medicine, Stanford, California, USA

Whitfield B. Growdon, MD
Division of Gynecologic Oncology, NYU Grossman
School of Medicine, New York, New York, USA

Oliver Dorigo, MD, PhD
Division of Gynecologic Oncology, Stanford University
School of Medicine, Stanford, California, USA

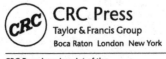

CRC Press
Taylor & Francis Group
Boca Raton London New York

CRC Press is an imprint of the
Taylor & Francis Group, an **informa** business

Second edition published 2023
by CRC Press
6000 Broken Sound Parkway NW, Suite 300, Boca Raton, FL 33487–2742

and by CRC Press
4 Park Square, Milton Park, Abingdon, Oxon, OX14 4RN

CRC Press is an imprint of Taylor & Francis Group, LLC

© 2023 Malte Renz, Elisabeth J. Diver, Whitfield B. Growdon, and Oliver Dorigo

Library of Congress Cataloging-in-Publication Data
Names: Renz, Malte, author. | Diver, Elisabeth J., author. | Growdon,
    Whitfield B., author. | Dorigo, Oliver, author.
Title: Synopsis of key gynecologic oncology trials / Malte Renz, Elisabeth
    J. Diver, Whitfield B. Growdon, Oliver Dorigo.
Description: Second edition. | Boca Raton : CRC Press, 2023. | Includes bibliographical references and index.
Summary: "This revised and updated new edition of a best-selling text remains a fast and convenient overview of
    the clinical trials in gynecologic cancer treatment, outlining the evidence base of treatment decisions in uterine,
    ovarian, cervical, and vulvar cancers, and gestational trophoblastic neoplasia. Residents and fellows will find this
    book an indispensable reference, while practitioners will welcome it as a clarification of the evidence base for
    treatment options. *Gives a convenient summary of trials in Gynecologic Oncology *Supplies an invaluable
    revision primer for those undertaking certification *Provides a uniquely up-to-date resource"—Provided by
    publisher.
Identifiers: LCCN 2022024517 (print) | LCCN 2022024518 (ebook) | ISBN 9781032135335 (hardback) |
    ISBN 9781032135328 (paperback) | ISBN 9781003229711 (ebook)
Subjects: MESH: Genital Neoplasms, Female—therapy | Clinical Trials as Topic
Classification: LCC RC280.G5 (print) | LCC RC280.G5 (ebook) | NLM WP 145 |
    DDC 616.99/465—dc23/eng/20220826
LC record available at https://lccn.loc.gov/2022024517
LC ebook record available at https://lccn.loc.gov/2022024518

ISBN: 978-1-032-13533-5 (hbk)
ISBN: 978-1-032-13532-8 (pbk)
ISBN: 978-1-003-22971-1 (ebk)

DOI: 10.1201/9781003229711

Typeset in Times
by Apex CoVantage, LLC

Zwei Dinge sind zu unserer Arbeit nötig: Unermüdliche Ausdauer und die Bereitschaft, etwas, in das man viel Arbeit gesteckt hat, wieder wegzuwerfen.*

Albert Einstein (1879–1955)

---

* Two things are required for our job: untiring efforts and the willingness to throw away something into which we have put a lot of work.

Contents

Preface to the Second Edition

This second edition has been updated and expanded while keeping its concise format. The book is intended to provide reference and synopsis of the existing evidence for treatment decisions in gynecologic oncology. As such, it covers trials addressing treatment modalities for all gynecologic malignancies, including endometrial cancer, ovarian cancer, cervical cancer, vulvar cancer, and gestational trophoblastic neoplasia.

I believe that this synopsis may help approach the ever-growing field of gynecologic oncology, learn about its diverse treatment options, apply them in the clinical setting, and identify areas of need for further clinical research. Thereby, this book illustrates the breadth of gynecologic oncology, which permits gynecologic oncologists to provide continuity of care and longitudinal follow-up for their patients through all stages of the disease.

Malte Renz
Palo Alto, California

Uterine Malignancies

1

1.1 ENDOMETRIAL CARCINOMA

1.1.1 Studies Addressing Surgical Treatment

Study: GOG 33

- **Citation:** (Creasman et al., 1987)
- **Highlight:** Study results led to surgical FIGO staging in 1988, which replaced the clinical FIGO staging from 1971
- **Design:**
  - Between 1977 and 1983: 621 patients with clinical stage I endometrial cancer enrolled
  - To assess risk of extrauterine spread, specifically spread to lymph nodes (LNs) and evaluate risk factors
- **Results:**
  - 22% with extrauterine spread
  - Overall 11% with LN metastases
    - 6% (36/621) with only pelvic lymph node (PLN) metastases
    - 3% (22/621) with PLN and para-aortic lymph node (PALN) metastases
    - 2% (12/621) with isolated PALN
    - 22/58 (38%) with positive PLN have positive PALN
  - Demonstrated relationship between tumor grade/depth of invasion and nodal disease
    - G1/endometrium only: 0%/0% with positive PLN/PALN
    - G1/outer third: 11%/6%
    - G2/endometrium only: 3%/3%
    - G2/outer third: 19%/14%
    - G3/endometrium only: 0%/0%
    - G3/outer third: 34%/23%
  - Defined additional risk factors
    - LVSI: Fourfold increased risk of positive LN
    - Intraperitoneal disease (positive peritoneal washings, adnexal metastasis, and extrauterine spread)

Study: GOG LAP2 trial

- **Citation:** (Walker et al., 2009)
- **Highlight:** Surgical approach: Compare laparoscopy (LSC) with exploratory laparotomy (exlap) for comprehensive surgical staging
- **Design:**
    - 2:1 randomization of 2,616 patients with clinical stage I to IIA endometrial cancer to open (n = 920) vs. laparoscopic surgery (n = 1,696), including hysterectomy/ salpingo-oophorectomy/ pelvic cytology/ pelvic and para-aortic lymphadenectomy (predominantly laparoscopic-assisted vaginal hysterectomy)
- **Results:**
    - LSC staging completed in 74.2% (conversion in 26%)
    - Conversion due to
        - Poor visibility: 14.6%
        - Metastatic cancer: 4.1%
        - Bleeding: 2.9%
    - Fewer moderate-to-severe postoperative AEs: 14% vs. 21% (LSC vs. exlap)
    - Similar rates of intraoperative complications
    - Longer OR time: 204 vs. 130 minutes
    - Fewer hospitalizations >2 days: 52% vs. 94%
    - LNs not removed in 8% vs. 4%
    - No difference in overall detection of advanced disease: 17% vs. 17%
    - 0.24% port-side metastasis
- **Conclusion:**
    - Laparoscopic staging feasible and safe regarding short-term outcomes

Study: GOG LAP2 trial

- **Citation:** (Walker et al., 2012)
- **Highlight:** Long-term follow-up
- **Design:**
    - Primary objective non-inferiority for recurrence (no more than 40% increased risk)
- **Results:**
    - Median follow-up: 59 months
    - Estimated HR for LSC: 1.14 (CI = 0.92–1.46); did not meet predefined criteria of non-inferiority
    - Estimated 3-yr recurrence rates: 11.39% vs. 10.24% (LSC vs. exlap); difference of 1.14% (less than 5.3% difference thought to show non-inferiority at time of study design)
    - 5-yr OS: 89.8% for both
- **Conclusion:**
    - Superior short-term outcomes as reported previously
    - Potential for increased risk of cancer recurrence with LSC vs. exlap quantified and small

1.1.1.1 Lymph Node Assessment

Study: A Study in the Treatment of Endometrial Cancer (ASTEC)—Surgical trial

- **Citation:** (ASTEC study group et al., 2009b)
- **Highlight:** No therapeutic benefit of routine lymphadenectomy
- **Design:**
  - 1998–2005: 1,408 patients with preoperative stage I endometrial carcinoma randomized to surgery with or without pelvic lymphadenectomy
  - To control for postsurgical treatment, patients with early-stage disease at intermediate or high risk of recurrence randomized (independent of LN status) into ASTEC radiotherapy trial
    - That is, randomized to observation or pelvic radiation if G3, serous, or clear cell; >50% myometrial invasion; or endocervical glandular invasion (IIA); nodal status did not alter use of radiation
- **Results:**
  - Median follow-up: 37 months
  - Absolute difference in OS: 1% in favor of standard surgery (study was designed to show improved OS by 10%)
  - Absolute difference in RFS: 6% in favor of standard surgery
- **Conclusion:**
  - → No evidence of benefit; pelvic lymphadenectomy cannot be recommended as routine procedure for therapeutic purposes
- **Discussion:**
  - Criticism
    - Absence of treatment in patients with positive nodes
    - Vaginal brachytherapy (VBT) permitted regardless of pelvic RT assignment based on institutional preference
    - Limited power
    - Poor quality of lymph node dissection (LND) (8% of patients in the LND group did not receive LND; 12% had <5 LN removed)
    - Absence of para-aortic lymph node dissection (PALND)
    - Lack of quality-of-life assessment
    - Overrepresentation of low-risk patients
    - However, next to CONSORT, only level 1 evidence on role of LND

Study: CONSORT (Consolidated Standards of Reporting Trials)

- **Citation:** (Benedetti Panici et al., 2008)
- **Highlight:** No therapeutic benefit of routine lymphadenectomy
- **Design:**
  - 1996–2006: 514 patients with preoperative stage I endometrial carcinoma randomized to surgery with or without pelvic lymphadenectomy
  - Required to have myometrial invasion; on intraoperative assessment, G1 and <50% myometrial invasion excluded from trial

- **Results:**
  - Median number of LN removed: 30
  - PALND at surgeon's discretion done in 26%
  - Postoperative therapy not prescribed but more common in the LND group (25% vs. 17%)
  - More early and late postoperative complications
  - Improved surgical staging: Positive LN found in 13.3% vs. 3.2%
  - 5-yr disease-free and OS similar with 81% and 85.9% (in the LND group) vs. 81.7% and 90% (in the no-LND group)
- **Conclusion:**
  - → No evidence of benefit; pelvic lymphadenectomy cannot be recommended as routine procedure for therapeutic purposes
- **Discussion:**
  - Criticism
    - No prescribed adjuvant therapy
    - Limited power
    - PALND at discretion
    - Lack of quality-of-life assessment
    - Overrepresentation of low-risk patients

Study: Mayo criteria—Retrospective

- **Citation** (Mariani et al., 2000b; Mariani et al., 2008)
- **Highlight:** Define criteria for patients at low risk for LN metastasis: G1, G2, ≤50% myometrial invasion, and tumor size ≤2 cm
- **Objective:** To define intraoperative pathological criteria based on frozen section to define a subgroup that will not require LND or adjuvant RT because of low risk of nodal disease and high disease-free survival (DFS)
- **Design:**
  - Retrospective study of 328 patients with G1 or 2, ≤50% myometrial invasion, and no intraoperative evidence of spread
- **Results:**
  - PLND performed in 57% (187); in 5% (9/187), positive LN found
  - Adjuvant RT administered to 20%
  - OS and RFS: 97% and 96%
  - Primary tumor diameter and lymphatic or vascular invasion affected longevity
  - No patient with tumor size ≤2 cm had positive LN or died

Study: Mayo criteria—Prospective

- **Citation:** (Mariani et al., 2008)
- **Highlight:** Define criteria for patients at low risk for LN metastasis: G1, G2, ≤50% myometrial invasion, and tumor size ≤2 cm

- **Design:**
  - Prospective study with 422 consecutive patients managed by predefined surgical guidelines differentiating low risk from at risk for dissemination
- **Results:**
  - 27% of all patients and 33% of endometrioid cases qualified as low risk
  - 20% of low-risk endometrioid cases had LND and negative LN
  - 22% (63/281) with risk factors and undergoing LND had positive LNs
    - Of patients with positive LNs, both PLN and PALN in 51%, only PLN in 33%, isolated PALN in 16% → 67% with lymphatic spread had positive PALNs
    - Of patients with positive PALNs, 77% with positive LN above the inferior mesenteric artery (IMA)
    - 28% with metastatic involvement of gonadal veins
- **Conclusion:**
  - → High rate of positive LNs above the IMA indicates need for systematic pelvic and para-aortic lymphadenectomy (vs. sampling) (with consideration of excising gonadal veins)

Study: Mayo experience with systematic PALND

- **Citation:** (Mariani et al., 2000a)
- **Highlight:** Systematic PALND
- **Design:**
  - Retrospective study
  - Group 1: 137 patients at high risk for para-aortic (PA) nodal disease
    - >50% myometrial invasion
    - Palpable positive pelvic nodes
    - Positive adnexa
  - Group 2: 51 patients with positive PLN or PALN
  - Compared with pelvic and para-aortic lymph node dissection (PPALND) and without (defined as dissection of ≥5 PALN)
- **Results:**
  - No difference in percentage who received postoperative extended field radiation
  - Group 1: 5-yr PFS and OS: 77% and 85% vs. 62% and 71% (complete PPALND vs. without)
  - Group 2: 5-yr PFS and OS: 76% and 77% vs. 36% and 42%
  - LN recurrences: 0% vs. 37%
  - Multivariate analysis: PPALND = predictor of PFS and OS (OR = 0.26 and 0.23; $p = 0.01$ and $p = 0.006$, respectively)
- **Conclusion:**
  - → Results suggest potential therapeutic role of PPALND in endometrial cancer

Study: SEPAL study (Survival Effect of Para-Aortic Lymphadenectomy)

- **Citation:** (Todo et al., 2010)
- **Design:**
  - Retrospective study of 671 patients treated in two different centers in Japan, matched for tumor type, grade, and stage
  - Complete pelvic lymphadenectomy vs. combined pelvic and para-aortic lymphadenectomy
  - If at intermediate or high risk (G1 and 2 if positive LVSI and IB, G3, non-endometrioid), for recurrence offered RT or CT
- **Results:**
  - OS longer in PPALND group; HR 0.53; CI = 0.38–0.76 (p = 0.0005)
  - OS longer in 407 patients at intermediate or high risk (p = 0.0009), independent of adjuvant therapy
  - But no improved OS in low-risk patients
  - In multivariate analysis: PPALND reduced risk of death compared to PLND (HR 0.44; CI = 0.30–0.64; p = <0.0001)
  - 328 patients at intermediate or high risk treated with adjuvant RT or CT: Survival improved with PPALND and with adjuvant CT, independently of another
- **Conclusion:**
  - → PPALND recommended for treatment of patients with endometrial cancer at intermediate or high risk of recurrence

Study: SENTI-ENDO (Sentinel Node and Endometrial Cancer)

- **Citation:** (Ballester et al., 2011)
- **Highlight:** SLN assessment
- **Design:**
  - 125 patients from nine centers in France with stage I–II endometrial cancer underwent pelvic SLN assessment with dual cervical injection (technetium and patent blue) and systematic PLND
- **Results:**
  - At least one SLN detected in 111/125 (88.8%)
  - Bilateral mapping: 77/125 (62%)
  - 19/111 (17%) with LN metastasis; 16 detected by SLN biopsy
  - For hemipelvis: NPV 100%; sensitivity 100%
  - For patient: NPV 97%, sensitivity 84% (two patients with metastatic LN contralateral; one in PA region; all type II endometrial carcinoma), and false-negative rate 6%
  - IHC and serial sectioning detected nine patients undiagnosed by hematoxylin and eosin (HE) (9/19 = 47%)
  - SLN biopsy upstaged 10% of patients with low-risk and 15% with intermediate-risk endometrial cancer

- **Conclusion:**
  - → SLN biopsy could be a trade-off between systematic lymphadenectomy and no dissection in patients with low and intermediate risk, and it could provide important data to tailor adjuvant therapy

Study: FIRES study (Fluorescence Imaging for Robotic Endometrial Sentinel Lymph Node Biopsy)

- **Citation:** (Rossi et al., 2017)
- **Highlight:** SLN assessment
- **Design:**
  - Eligible patients with clinical stage I endometrial cancer of all grades and histologies undergoing robotic staging surgery
  - Cervical injection of indocyanine
  - SLN mapping followed by PLND with or without PALND
  - Negative SLN by HE ultra-staging with IHC for cytokeratin
- **Results:**
  - Between August 2012 and October 2015: SLN biopsy and complete PLND performed in 340 patients and PALND in 196 patients
  - 86% (293/340) with successful mapping of at least one SLN
  - Bilateral mapping: 52%
  - 41 (12%) patients with positive LNs; 36/41 with at least one mapped LN
  - Nodal metastasis identified in 35/36 patients
  - Sensitivity of SLN 97.2% (35/36 patients), NPV 99.6%, and false-negative rate (1-sensitivity) 2.8%
- **Conclusion:**
  - → SLN mapping with indocyanine green with high diagnostic accuracy
  - SLN mapping can safely replace LND in staging of endometrial cancer
  - SLN mapping will not identify 3% of patients with nodal disease but expose fewer patients to morbidity of complete LND

Study: SENTOR trial (Sentinel Lymph Node Biopsy vs. Lymphadenectomy for Intermediate- and High-Grade Endometrial Cancer Staging)

- **Citation:** (Cusimano et al., 2021)
- **Highlight:** SLN in high-grade endometrial cancer
- **Design:**
  - Prospective cohort study of 156 patients with stage I grade 2 endometrioid or high-grade endometrial cancer underwent SLN injection and biopsy and backup lymphadenectomy; for grade 2 endometrioid endometrial cancer pelvic lymphadenectomy and for high-grade endometrial cancer pelvic and para-aortic lymphadenectomy
- **Results:**
  - 126/156 with high-grade endometrial cancer

- All underwent pelvic lymphadenectomy; 80% also para-aortic lymphadenectomy
- SLN detection rate: 97.4% per patient, 87.5% per hemipelvis, and 77.6% bilaterally
- 26/27 with nodal metastasis correctly identified by SLN; sensitivity 96%; false-negative rate 4%
- 2/27 with single metastatic SLN outside the PLN boundaries (one parametrial and one common iliac); 5/27 required IHC for diagnosis
- **Conclusion:**
  - → SLN is a viable option for surgical staging of endometrial cancer

1.1.2 Studies Addressing Adjuvant Therapy

1.1.2.1 Radiation

Study: GOG 99

- **Citation:** (Keys et al., 2004)
- **Highlight:** Pelvic RT for high intermediate-risk group
- **Design:**
  - 392 patients with intermediate risk (IB, IC, IIA [occult], and IIB [occult]) randomized after surgery (including PLND and possibly PALND) to EBRT vs. observation
  - Intermediate risk defined based on GOG 33
    - IB, IC, IIA (occult), and IIB (occult) (i.e., any degree of myometrial invasion, any grade, and no evidence of LN involvement)
    - Expected 5-yr recurrence rate: 20–25%, almost all within 24 months
- **Results:**
  - Median follow-up: 69 months
  - Adjuvant EBRT reduced estimated cumulative incidence of recurrences: 12% vs. 3% (observation vs. EBRT)
  - Particularly in 'high-intermediate risk' group: 26% vs. 6%
  - GOG 99 defined high-intermediate risk
    - (Predictive of local and distant recurrence; 2/3 of all recurrences in those patients with high intermediate risk [HIR] features)
    - HIR: Patient age and any of the following
      - Grade 2 or 3
      - LVSI
      - Outer third myometrial invasion
      - >70 and one risk factor, 50–69 and two risk factors, and >18 and all three risk factors
  - However, estimated 4-yr OS: 86% vs. 92% (p = 0.557) (observation vs. EBRT)
  - 4-yr disease-specific survival
    - All: 92% vs. 95%

- In HIR: 83% vs. 90%; CI: 0.29–1.24
- In low/intermediate risk: 98% vs. 98%
- **Conclusion:**
  - → EBRT reduces recurrences but should be limited to HIR patients

Study: PORTEC-1 (Postoperative Radiation Therapy for Endometrial Cancer)

- **Citation:** (Creutzberg et al., 2000)
- **Highlight:** RT in early-stage endometrial cancer
- **Design:**
  - 714 patients with stage I endometrial cancer (G1 with >50% myometrial invasion, G2 with any invasion, and G3 with superficial invasion <50%)—*no nodal assessment*—randomized to EBRT vs. observation
- **Results:**
  - Median follow-up: 52 months
  - 5-yr locoregional (i.e., vaginal, pelvic, or both) recurrence rate: 4% vs. 14% (p < 0.001) (EBRT vs. observation)
    - 73% vaginal recurrences
  - 5-yr OS: 81% vs. 85% (p = 0.31)
  - Endometrial cancer-related deaths: 9% vs. 6% (p = 0.37)
  - Complications: 25% vs. 6% (2/3 grade 1) (p < 0.0001)
  - 2-yr survival after vaginal recurrence: 79%; after pelvic recurrence/distant metastasis: 21%
  - Survival after relapse better in control group (p = 0.02)
  - Multivariate analysis: Age <60 and RT favorable prognostic factors
- **Conclusion:**
  - → EBRT reduces locoregional recurrences but did not increase OS and increases treatment-related complications
  - EBRT not indicated in stage I <60 yrs (except those with G3 and deep invasion because those are not represented in the study) and G2 with superficial invasion

Study: PORTEC-1

- **Citation:** (Creutzberg et al., 2011)
- **Highlight:** Long-term follow-up
- **Results:**
  - 15-yr locoregional recurrence: 5.8% vs. 15.5% (EBRT vs. observation)
  - 15-yr rate of distant metastasis: 9% vs. 7% (p = 0.25)
  - 15-yr OS: 52% vs. 60% (p = 0.14)
  - Failure-free survival: 50% vs. 54%
  - For HIR, 15-yr OS: 41% vs. 48% (p = 0.51)
    - Here, the authors define HIR: G3, age >60, and MI >50% (at least two out of three)
  - Second primary cancers: 22% vs. 16% (p = 0.1)

- Multivariate analysis confirmed prognostic significance of G3; age >60; MI >50%
- **Conclusion:**
  - → 15-yr long-term data confirm relevance of HIR criteria for treatment selection; EBRT should be avoided in low- and intermediate-risk patients
  - No OS benefit for adjuvant RT

Study: PORTEC-1

- **Citation:** (Nout et al., 2011)
- **Highlight:** Long-term follow-up and health-related quality of life (HRQOL)
- **Results:**
  - EBRT associated with 26% risk of adverse effects, mainly grade 1 and 2 GI toxicity
  - EBRT associated with long-term urinary and bowel symptoms and lower physical function even after 15 yrs
- **Conclusion:**
  - → EBRT justified only for patients at high risk for recurrence

Study: PORTEC-2

- **Citation:** (Nout et al., 2010)
- **Highlight:** VBT for HIR endometrial cancer
- **Design:**
  - 427 patients with stage I and IIA and HIR (*no nodal assessment!*) randomized to VBT (21 Gy high-dose rate [HDR] in three fractions, or 30 Gy low-dose rate [LDR]) vs. pelvic EBRT (46 Gy in 23 fractions)
  - Non-inferiority study with primary endpoint of vaginal recurrence
  - Here, HIR defined as (1) >60 *and* outer 1/3 myometrial invasion for G1 or 2 *or* middle third and G3, and (2) stage IIA, any age (no nodal assessment in this study) (different from definition in PORTEC-1 follow-up)
  - ↔ High risk excluded: Non-endometrioid cancer, stage IC G3, and stage IIB or higher
- **Results:**
  - Estimated 5-yr rate of vaginal recurrence: 1.8% vs. 1.6% (VBT vs. EBRT)
  - 5-yr rate locoregional relapse (vaginal or pelvic): 5.1% vs. 2.1% (p = 0.17)
  - Isolated pelvic recurrence: 1.5% vs. 0.5% (p = 0.3)
  - Distant metastasis: 8.3% vs. 5.7% (p = 0.46)
  - OS: 84.8% vs. 79.6% (p = 0.57)
  - DFS: 82.7% vs. 78.1%
  - Grade 1–2 GI toxicity significantly lower: 12.6% vs. 53.8%
- **Conclusion:**
  - → VBT should be adjuvant treatment of choice in HIR

Study: ASTEC/EN.5—Radiotherapy trial

- **Citation:** (ASTEC/EN.5 Study Group et al., 2009a)

- **Highlight:** EBRT for intermediate- or high-risk early-stage endometrial cancer
- **Background:**
  - ASTEC and EN.5 set up as individual trials to investigate pelvic RT in early-stage endometrial cancer at intermediate/high risk for recurrence
  - EN.5 started in 1996 in Canada; insufficient recruitment
  - In 1998, UK launched ASTEC and invited EN.5
  - Therefore, two trials with separate randomization to make one intergroup trial
  - 1996–2005: EBRT in early-stage endometrial cancer with intermediate or high risk of recurrence
- **Design:**
  - 905 patients randomized to EBRT (40–46 Gy in 20–25 fractions) vs. observation
  - Intermediate risk
    - Stages IA and IB G3
    - IC G1 and G2
    - IIA G1 and G2
  - High-risk early stage
    - IC and IIA G3
    - USC and clear-cell histology
  - Lymphadenectomy not required for randomization
  - VBT option in both arms
- **Results:**
  - Median follow-up: 58 months
  - 67 patients in EBRT group and 68 patients in observation group had died (HR 1.05; CI = 0.75–1.48; p = 0.77)
  - 5-yr OS in both groups: 84%
  - Combining data from ASTEC and EN.5, in meta-analysis of trials (HR 1.04; CI = 0.84–1.29)
  - With VBT used in 53% of patients in ASTEC/EN.5; local recurrence rate in the observation group at 5 yrs: 6.1%
- **Discussion:**
  - → EBRT cannot be recommended as routine in intermediate- or high-risk early-stage endometrial cancer patients
  - Absolute benefit of EBRT in preventing isolated local recurrences small and not without toxicity

1.1.2.2 Chemoradiation

Study: RTOG 9708 (Radiation Therapy Oncology Group)

- **Citation:** (Greven et al., 2004; Greven et al., 2006)
- **Highlight:** Chemoradiation
- **Design:**
  - Phase II trial: 46 patients with completely resected high-risk endometrial cancer received chemoradiation therapy (CTRT)

- G2 or 3 with >50% myometrial invasion, cervical stroma invasion, or pelvic confined extrauterine disease
- Patients received pelvic RT (45 Gy in 25 fractions) with cisplatin (50 mg/m^2) on days 1 and 28; VBT after EBRT with low-dose-rate or high-dose-rate applicator, then 4 C of cisplatin (50 mg/m^2) and paclitaxel (175 mg/m^2) q 4 wks)
- **Results:**
  - At 4 yrs, regional, pelvic, and distant recurrence rates: 2%, 2%, and 19%
  - OS at 4 yrs: 85%; for stage III: 77%
  - DFS at 4 yrs: 81%; for stage III: 72%
  - No recurrences for stages IC, IIA, and IIB
- **Conclusion:**
  - → Local control excellent (suggesting additive effect of CT and RT); distant metastases continue to occur in advanced stage

Study: PORTEC-3

- **Citation:** (de Boer et al., 2018)
- **Highlight:** CTRT cannot be recommended for stage I + II, but should be considered for stage III
- **Design:**
  - 660 patients randomized to adjuvant CT during and after radiation therapy (CTRT) vs. RT alone in high-risk endometrial cancer
    - Stage I: G3 endometrioid with deep myometrial invasion and/or LVSI
    - Stage II or III: Endometrioid
    - Stage I–III: Serous or clear cell
  - CTRT: EBRT plus 2 C cisplatin 50 mg/m^2 on days 1 and 22 of RT, followed by 4 C carboplatin AUC 5 and paclitaxel 175 mg/m^2 q 3 wks
  - RT: EBRT (48.6 Gy in 1.8 fractions)
- **Results:**
  - Median follow-up: 60.2 months
  - 5-yr OS: 81.8% vs. 76.7% (HR: 0.76; CI: 0.54–1.06; p = 0.11) (CTRT vs. RT)
  - 5-yr FFS: 75.5% vs. 68.6% (HR: 0.71; CI: 0.53–0.95; p = 0.022)
    - Stage III endometrial cancer
      - 5-yr OS: 78.7% vs. 69.8% (p = 0.13; adjusted p = 0.074)
      - 5-yr FFS: 69.3% vs. 58% (p = 0.031; adjusted p = 0.014)
  - ≥Grade 3 AEs: 60% vs. 12% (p < 0.0001)
  - More toxicity and lower quality of life with CTRT, especially early on
  - >Grade 2 persistent neuropathy: 8% vs. 1% at 3 yrs (p < 0.0001)
- **Conclusion:**
  - → Adjuvant CT during and after radiotherapy for high-risk endometrial cancer did not improve 5-yr OS but FFS
  - In view of high recurrence risk for stage III endometrial cancer, CTRT should be considered

Study: PORTEC-3

- **Citation:** (de Boer et al., 2016)
- **Highlight:** Quality of life
- **Results:**
  - Despite increased physician- and patient-reported toxicities, CT given during and after RT in patients with high-risk endometrial cancer feasible
  - Rapid recovery after treatment
  - Persistence of patient-reported sensory neurological symptoms in 25%

Study: PORTEC-3

- **Citation:** (Leon-Castillo et al., 2020)
- **Highlight:** Molecular classification
- **Background:** The Cancer Genome Atlas (TCGA) defined an endometrial cancer classification with high prognostic value. Studied here prognosis and impact of CT for each molecular subgroup.
- **Design:**
  - IHC on paraffin-embedded tissues of 423 patients for p53, mismatch repair (MMR) proteins, and DNA sequencing for *POLE* exonuclease domain
- **Results:**
  - Molecular analysis successful in 410 high-risk endometrial cancers identified four subgroups
    - p53abn (n = 93; 23%)
    - *POLE*-mut (n = 51; 12%)
    - MMRd (n = 137; 33%)
    - No specific molecular profile (NSMP; n = 129; 32%)
  - 5-yr RFS
    - p53abn: 48%
      - 59% vs. 36% (chemoRT vs. RT)
    - *POLE*-mut: 98%
      - 100% vs. 97%
    - MMRd: 72%
      - 68% vs. 76%
    - NSMP: 74%
      - 80% vs. 68%
- **Conclusion:**
  - → Molecular classification with strong prognostic value in high-risk endometrial cancer regardless of histology; significantly improved RFS with adjuvant chemoRT for p53abn cancers

Study: PORTEC-4a

- **Citation:** NCT03469674; ongoing
- **Highlight:** Molecular profile-based adjuvant treatment

- **Design:**
  - Randomized 2:1 to molecular-integrated risk profile-based adjuvant treatment (VBT, external beam radiotherapy, or observation) vs. adjuvant VBT

Study: GOG 249 (RTOG 1070 endorsed)

- **Citation:** (Randall et al., 2019)
- **Highlight:** Adjuvant pelvic RT (PXRT) vs. vaginal cuff brachytherapy plus CT (VCB/C) for high-risk early-stage endometrial cancer
- **Design:**
  - 601 patients randomized to VBT followed by 3 C paclitaxel 175 mg/m^2 and carboplatin AUC 6 q 3 wks vs. pelvic RT (45–50 Gy in 28 fractions; optional vaginal cuff boost for stage II and stage I USC or clear-cell histology)
    - Endometrial cancer with HIR factors as defined by GOG-33
    - Stage II
    - USC or clear cell stage I–II
- **Results:**
  - 74% with stage I
  - 71% endometrioid, 15% serous, and 5% clear cell
  - Median follow-up: 53 months
  - No difference in RFS and OS
    - 5-yr RFS: 0.76 vs. 0.76 (PXRT vs. VCB/C)
    - 5-yr OS: 0.87 vs. 0.85
  - Vaginal (2.5%) and distant (18%) recurrence rates similar with HR 1.0, respectively
  - Pelvic and para-aortic nodal recurrence at 5 yrs: 4% vs. 9% (HR: 0.47; CI = 0.24–0.94)
  - AEs
    - More short-term complications in VCB/C
    - Long-term complications similar
- **Conclusion:**
  - → Superiority of VCB/C compared to PXRT not demonstrated; PXRT remains effective, well tolerated, and appropriate adjuvant treatment in high-risk early-stage endometrial carcinomas of all histologies

Study: GOG 258

- **Citation:** (Matei et al., 2019)
- **Highlight:** CTRT vs. CT
- **Design:**
  - Between June 2009 and July 2014; 707 patients with stage III and IVA (<2 cm residual disease) or stage I/II serous or clear-cell endometrial cancer *and* positive cytology randomized to cisplatin 50 mg/m^2 on days

1 and 29 with volume-directed radiation (45 Gy +/− brachytherapy) followed by carboplatin AUC 5 and paclitaxel 175 mg/m^2 q 3 wks for 4 C and G-CSF support (C-RT) vs. carboplatin AUC 6 and paclitaxel 175 mg/m^2 q 3 wks for 6 C (CT)

- **Results:**
  - Median follow-up: 47 months
  - Similar toxicity
    - ≥Grade 3 AEs: 58% vs. 63% (C-RT vs. CT)
  - 5-yr RFS: 59% vs. 58% (HR 0.9; CI = 0.74–1.1)
    - Vaginal recurrences: 2% vs. 7% (HR 0.36; CI = 0.16–0.82)
    - Pelvic/para-aortic recurrences: 11% vs. 20% (HR: 0.43; CI = 0.28–0.66)
    - Distant metastases: 27% vs. 21% (HR 1.36; CI = 1–1.86)
- **Conclusion:**
  - → C-RT was not associated with longer RFS than CT alone

1.1.2.3 Chemotherapy

- **Background:** Initial combination: cyclophosphamide and doxorubicin, then cyclophosphamide, doxorubicin, and cisplatin; however, no benefit for triple regimen over doxorubicin and cisplatin

Study: GOG 107

- **Citation:** (Thigpen et al., 2004)
- **Highlight:** Cisplatin + doxorubicin
- **Design:**
  - 281 chemo-naïve patients with stage III or IV endometrial cancer or recurrent disease randomized to doxorubicin 60 mg/m^2 q 3 wks vs. doxorubicin 60 mg/m^2 plus cisplatin 50 mg/m^2 q 3 wks until disease progression or total of 500 mg/m^2 doxorubicin
- **Results:**
  - ORR: 42% vs. 25% (combination vs. doxorubicin alone)
  - Median PFS: 5.7 vs. 3.8 months
  - Median OS: 9 vs. 9.2 months
  - More grade 3–4 leukopenia, thrombocytopenia, anemia, and nausea/vomiting for combination
- **Conclusion:**
  - → Adding cisplatin to doxorubicin in advanced endometrial cancer improves ORR and PFS with negligible impact on OS and increased toxicity

Study: GOG 163

- **Citation:** (Fleming et al., 2004b)
- **Highlight:** Doxorubicin + paclitaxel

- **Design:**
  - 317 chemo-naïve patients with stage III or IV endometrial cancer or recurrent disease randomized to doxorubicin 60 mg/m^2 q 3 wks and cisplatin 50 mg/m^2 q 3 wks × 7 C vs. doxorubicin 60 mg/m^2 q 3 wks and paclitaxel 150 mg/m^2 over 24 hrs plus filgrastim q 3 wks for 7 C
- **Results:**
  - No significant difference in response rate (40% vs. 43%); PFS (7.2 vs. 6 months) or OS (12.6 vs. 13.6 months)
  - Similar toxicities
- **Conclusion:**
  - → Doxorubicin and 24-hr paclitaxel plus filgrastim not superior to doxorubicin and cisplatin

Study: GOG 177

- **Citation:** (Fleming et al., 2004a)
- **Highlight:** Cisplatin + doxorubicin +/– paclitaxel (AP vs. TAP)
- **Design:**
  - 263 chemo-naïve patients with stage III or IV endometrial cancer or recurrent disease randomized to doxorubicin 60 mg/m^2 and cisplatin 50 mg/m^2 q 3 wks × 7 C (AP) +/– paclitaxel 160 mg/m^2 on day 2 plus filgrastim (TAP) for 7 C q 3 wks
- **Results:**
  - ORR: 57% vs. 34% (TAP vs. AP) (p < 0.01)
  - PFS: 8.3 vs. 5.3 months (p < 0.01)
  - OS: 15.3 vs. 12.3 months (p < 0.037)
  - Grade 3 and 2 peripheral neuropathy: 12 and 27% vs. 1 and 4%
  - Neutropenic fever: 3% vs. 2%
- **Conclusion:**
  - → TAP significantly improves ORR, PFS, and OS (caveat: peripheral neuropathy)

Study: GOG 184

- **Citation:** (Homesley et al., 2009)
- **Highlight:** Chemoradiation with cisplatin/ doxorubicin +/– paclitaxel
- **Design:**
  - 552 patients with stage III or IV and postoperative maximal 2 cm residual disease randomized after RT to CT with or without paclitaxel
  - 6 C cisplatin and doxorubicin with or without paclitaxel (160 mg/m^2) (i.e., CD and DCP); initially, only paclitaxel patients received granulocyte growth factor, then after 2002 all patients
  - RT: pelvic EBRT (50.4 Gy in 28 fractions) and para-aortic fields (43.5 Gy); optional intravaginal boost (7 Gy HDR in one fraction, or 10 Gy LDR)
- **Results:**
  - Hematologic AEs, sensory neuropathy, and myalgia more frequent and severe in CDP (p < 0.01)

- OS and PFS at 36 months: 62% vs. 64% (CD vs. CDP)
- In a subgroup analysis, CDP with 50% reduction of recurrence or death among patients with gross residual disease
- **Conclusion:**
  - → Addition of paclitaxel not associated with significant improvement in RFS, but increased toxicity

Study: GOG 122

- **Citation:** (Homesley et al., 2009; Randall et al., 2006)
- **Highlight:** Whole-abdominal irradiation
- **Design:**
  - 396 chemo-naïve patients with stage III or IV endometrial cancer and maximum 2 cm postoperative residual disease randomized to whole-abdominal irradiation 30 Gy in 20 fractions with a 15 Gy boost vs. doxorubicin 60 mg/m^2 and cisplatin 50 mg/m^2 q 3 wks × 7 C
- **Results:**
  - 50% with endometrioid endometrial cancer
  - HR for progression adjusted for stage: 0.71 favoring CT (p < 0.01)
  - HR for death adjusted for stage: 0.68 favoring CT (p < 0.01)
- **Conclusion:**
  - → CT significantly improved PFS and OS

Study: GOG 209

- **Citation:** (Miller et al., 2020)
- **Highlight:** Paclitaxel + carboplatin (TC) vs. paclitaxel + cisplatin + doxorubicin (TAP)
- **Design:**
  - 1,381 chemo-naïve patients with stage III or IV or recurrent endometrial cancer randomized in non-inferiority trial to doxorubicin 45 mg/m^2 and cisplatin 50 mg/m^2 followed by paclitaxel 160 mg/m^2 on day 2 with growth factor support (TAP) q 3 wks for 7 C vs. paclitaxel 175 mg/m^2 and carboplatin AUC 6 (TC) q 3 wks for 7 C
- **Results:**
  - Non-inferiority concluded for
    - Median OS: 37 vs. 41 months (HR 1.002; CI = 0.9–1.12) (TC vs. TAP)
    - Median PFS: 13 vs. 14 months
  - >Grade 2 sensory neuropathy: 20% vs. 26%
  - Thrombocytopenia: 12% vs. 23%
  - However, neutropenia: 80% vs. 52%
  - Neutropenic fever: 6% vs. 7%
  - 7 C completed in 69% vs. 63%
- **Conclusion:**
  - → TC not inferior in PFS and OS; TC global first-line standard for advanced endometrial cancer

1.1.3 Studies Addressing Treatment of Recurrent Endometrial Carcinoma

1.1.3.1 Hormonal Therapy

- **Background:** Endocrine therapy valuable, particularly in recurrent disease
  - Overall response to progestins 25%; higher dose does not increase effect
  - Problem: receptor downregulation → tamoxifen recruits progesterone receptors

Study: Fiorica study

- **Citation:** (Fiorica et al., 2004)
- **Highlight:** Alternating megestrol acetate + tamoxifen
- **Design:**
  - Phase II trial: 56 patients with recurrent or advanced endometrial cancer without prior cytotoxic or hormonal treatment received megestrol acetate 80 mg BID × 3 wks followed by tamoxifen 20 mg BID × 3 wks; alternating sequence continued until progression or toxicity
- **Results:**
  - ORR: 27% (12 CR; 3 PR), in 8/15 duration of response >20 months
    - ORR: 38% in G1, 24% in G2, and 22% in G3
    - ORR: Extra pelvic disease 31% vs. 14% pelvic/vaginal disease
    - PFS: 2.7 months
    - OS: 14.0 months
- **Conclusion:**
  - → Regimen of alternating megestrol acetate and tamoxifen is active and may result in prolonged CR in some patients

Study: GOG 248

- **Citation:** (Fleming et al., 2014c)
- **Highlight:** Temsirolimus +/− megestrol acetate/tamoxifen
- **Design:**
  - Phase II trial: 71 patients with stage III or IV or persistent or recurrent endometrial cancer after up to one prior CT randomized to temsirolimus 25 mg q wk and megestrol acetate 80 mg BID × 3 wks alternating with tamoxifen 20 mg BID × 3 wks vs. temsirolimus 25 mg q wk alone
    - Temsirolimus: Mammalian target of rapamycin (mTOR) inhibitor
- **Results:**
  - Combination arm closed early because of excess deep vein thrombosis (five) and pulmonary embolism (two)
  - 3/21 (14%) responses in combination arm
  - 11/50 (22%) responses in single-drug arm (3 CR; 8 PR)
    - With prior CT, ORR: 24%

- – Without prior CT, ORR: 19%
- – 2/4 patients with clear-cell cancer responded
- **Conclusion:**
  - • → Adding megestrol/tamoxifen did not enhance activity and was associated with excess risk of venous thromboembolism
  - • Temsirolimus activity preserved in patients with prior CT

Study: Slomovitz study

- **Citation:** (Slomovitz et al., 2015)
- **Highlight:** Letrozole + everolimus
- **Background:**
  - • Resistance to hormonal treatment derived from the phosphoinositide 3-kinase (PI3-kinase) pathway may be overcome by targeting mTOR
- **Design:**
  - • Phase II trial: 35 patients with measurable disease and up to two prior lines received 10 mg everolimus qd + 2.5 mg letrozole qd
    - – Everolimus: mTOR inhibitor
- **Results:**
  - • CBR: 40%
  - • RR: 32% (9 CR; 2 PR)
  - • No treatment discontinuation because of toxicity
  - • Serous histology predictor of lack of response
  - • Endometrioid histology and beta-catenin mutations responded well
- **Conclusion:**
  - • Everolimus + letrozole results in high CBR and RR in recurrent endometrial cancer

Study: GOG 3007

- **Citation:** (Slomovitz et al., 2022)
- **Highlight:** Letrozole + everolimus vs. tamoxifen/medroxyprogesterone acetate
- **Design:**
  - • Phase II trial: 74 patients with measurable stage III + IV or recurrent endometrial with ≤1 systemic regimen randomized to 10 mg everolimus + letrozole 2.5 mg qd (EL) vs. 20 mg tamoxifen BID alternating weeks with 200 mg medroxyprogesterone acetate qd + 20 mg tamoxifen BID (MT)
- **Results:**
  - • Response rate: 22% vs. 25% (everolimus + letrozole vs. medroxyprogesterone acetate + tamoxifen)
    - – CR: 1 vs. 3
  - • Median PFS: 6 vs. 4 months
    - – Chemo-naïve: 28 vs. 5 months
    - – With prior CT: 4 vs. 3 months

- ≥Grade 3 AEs: Anemia (24% vs. 6%), mucositis (5% vs. 0%), and thromboembolic events (0% vs. 11%)
- **Conclusion:**
  - → EL and MT with meaningful efficacy in recurrent endometrial cancer

1.1.3.2 Chemotherapy

Study: GOG 129-C

- **Citation:** (Lincoln et al., 2003)
- **Highlight:** Single-agent paclitaxel
- **Design:**
  - 44 patients with persistent or recurrent endometrial cancer who failed prior CT received single-agent paclitaxel 200 mg/m^2 q 21 d or 175 mg/m^2 if prior pelvic RT
- **Results:**
  - CR: 3/44 (6.8%)
  - PR: 9/44 (20.5%)
  - ORR: 27.3%
  - Median number of paclitaxel cycles to response 2 and median duration of response 4.2 months
  - Median OS: 10.3 months
  - AEs
    - ≥Grade 3 or 4 neutropenia: 64% (28/44)
    - Grade 3 neurotoxicity: 9% (4/44)
    - ≥Grade 3 or 4 GI symptoms: 7% (3/44)
    - No cardiac toxicity
- **Conclusion:**
  - → Single-agent paclitaxel active in endometrial cancer after prior CT

Study: GOG 86P

- **Citation:** (Aghajanian et al., 2018)
- **Highlight:** Carboplatin + paclitaxel + bevacizumab (BEV)
- **Design:**
  - Phase II trial: 349 patients randomized to three arms for initial treatment of stage III or IVA, stage IVB, or recurrent endometrial cancer
    - Arm 1: Paclitaxel 175 mg/m^2, carboplatin AUC 6 + BEV 15 mg/kg q 3 wks × 6 C, followed by BEV maintenance 15 mg/kg q 3 wks
      - If prior RT: Paclitaxel reduced to 135 mg/m^2 and carboplatin to AUC 5
    - Arm 2: Paclitaxel 175 mg/m^2, carboplatin AUC 5 + temsirolimus 25 mg iv on days 1 and 8, followed by temsirolimus maintenance 25 mg iv on days 1, 8, and 15
      - If prior RT: Paclitaxel reduced to 135 mg/m^2 and temsirolimus to 20 mg iv

- Arm 3: Ixabepilone 30 mg/m^2, carboplatin AUC 6 + BEV 15 mg/kg q 3 wks × 6 C, followed by BEV maintenance 15 mg/kg q 3 wks
  - If prior RT: Ixabepilone reduced to 25 mg/m^2 and carboplatin to AUC 5
- Ixabepilone stabilizes microtubules, highly potent, retains activity in cases where tumor cells are insensitive to paclitaxel
- 1:1:1 randomization, stratified by measurable disease, recurrent disease, and prior pelvic RT
- GOG 209 used as historic control

- **Results:**
  - ORR: 59.5%, 55.3%, and 52.9%, compared to 51.2% (arm 1, 2, 3 vs. GOG 209)
  - PFS not significantly increased in any arm compared to historic control (p > 0.039)
  - OS significantly increased in arm 1 compared to historic control (p < 0.039) but not in arm 2 or 3
- **Conclusion:**
  - → PFS not increased; OS increased by combination paclitaxel/carboplatin/BEV relative to historic control

1.1.3.3 Targeted Therapy

Study: GOG 229E

- **Citation:** (Aghajanian et al., 2011)
- **Highlight:** Single-agent BEV
- **Design:**
  - Phase II trial: 52 patients with persistent or recurrent endometrial cancer after one to two prior cytotoxic regimens received BEV 15 mg/kg q 3 wks until progression or toxicity
- **Results:**
  - ORR: 13.5% (1 CR; 6 PR)
  - SD for 6 months: 40.4%
  - PFS: 4.2 months
  - OS: 10.5 months
- **Conclusion:**
  - → Single-agent BEV well tolerated and active in pretreated endometrial cancer

Study: GOG 229G

- **Citation:** (Alvarez et al., 2013)
- **Highlight:** BEV + temsirolimus
- **Design:**
  - Phase II trial: 49 patients with persistent or recurrent endometrial cancer after one to two prior cytotoxic regimens

- BEV 10 mg/kg every other week and temsirolimus 25 mg iv q wk until progression or toxicity
  - Temsirolimus: mTOR inhibitor
- **Results:**
  - Two GI perforations, two gastrointestinal–vaginal fistulas, one grade 4 thrombosis/embolism, and three treatment-related deaths
  - ORR: 24.5% (1 CR; 11 PR)
  - SD for 6 months: 46.9%
  - PFS: 5.6 months
  - OS: 16.9 months
- **Conclusion:**
  - → Combination deemed active but with significant toxicity

Study: Fader trial

- **Citation:** (Fader et al., 2018)
- **Highlight:** Trastuzumab in uterine serous carcinoma
- **Background:**
  - ↔ GOG-181B (Fleming et al., 2017): Single-agent trastuzumab in advanced/recurrent endometrial cancer; failed to reach target accrual and deemed inactive (only 47% of patients had ultimately HER2/neu gene amplification)
- **Design:**
  - Multicenter phase II trial from 2011 to 2017: 58 patients with primary stage III or IV or recurrent HER2/neu-positive endometrial cancer randomized to carboplatin/paclitaxel +/– trastuzumab
  - Carboplatin AUC 5, paclitaxel 175 mg/m^2 over 3 hrs q 3 wks × 6 C (co) vs. carboplatin AUC 5, paclitaxel 175 mg/m^2 over 3 hrs + trastuzumab 8 mg/kg for first dose and 6 mg/kg for subsequent cycles q 3 wks × 6 C followed by trastuzumab 6 mg/kg maintenance until progression or toxicity
  - In recurrent disease and prior doxorubicin or doxil treatment, patients may not have ≥320 mg/m^2 total dose and normal baseline ECHO
  - Trastuzumab: Humanized monoclonal antibody against human epidermal growth factor 2 HER2/neu
  - HER2/neu overexpressed in 30% of uterine serous carcinomas
    - Specimen required to contain ≥10% USC
    - HER2/neu positivity: IHC 3+, or 2+ with gene amplification confirmed by FISH
    - Patients may have undergone optimal or suboptimal primary surgery
- **Results:**
  - All 58 patients
    - PFS: 8.0 vs. 12.6 months (HR: 0.44; CI: 0.26–0.76; p = 0.005) (co vs. exp)
  - 41 patients with primary stage III or IV
    - PFS: 9.3 vs. 17.9 months (HR: 0.4; CI 0.2–0.8; p = 0.013)

- 17 patients with recurrent disease
  - PFS: 6.0 vs. 9.2 months (HR: 0.14; CI 0.04–0.53; p = 0.003)
- No difference in toxicity between arms
- **Conclusion:**
  - → Addition of trastuzumab to carboplatin/ paclitaxel well tolerated and increased PFS

Study: MITO END-2

- **Citation:** (Lorusso et al., 2019)
- **Highlight:** Carbo/Taxol +/– BEV
- **Design:**
  - In phase II trial: 108 patients with stage III–IV or recurrent endometrial cancer randomized to carboplatin AUC 5 + paclitaxel 175 mg/m^2 vs. carboplatin AUC 5 + paclitaxel 175 mg/m^2 plus 15 mg/kg BEV (combination and maintenance)
- **Results:**
  - ORR: 53.1% vs. 74.4% (without vs. with bev)
  - Median PFS: 10.5 vs. 13.7 months; HR 0.84; p = 0.43
  - Median OS: 29.7 vs. 40 months; HR 0.71; p = 0.24
  - 6-month DCR: 70.4% vs. 90.7%
  - ≥2 grade AEs: Hypertension (0% vs. 21%), thromboembolic events (2% vs. 11%)
- **Conclusion:**
  - → BEV combined with CT in advanced/recurrent endometrial cancer failed to show significant increase in PFS

1.1.3.4 Immunotherapy

Study: Keynote-16

- **Citation:** (Le et al., 2015)
- **Highlight:** Pembrolizumab in mismatch repair (MMR) deficient solid tumors
- **Design:**
  - Phase 2 trial: 41 patients with progressive metastatic colorectal cancers with and without MMR deficiency and non-colorectal cancers with MMR deficiency
  - Pembrolizumab: Programmed cell death protein-1 (PD-1) antibody
  - 10 mg/kg iv pembrolizumab q 14 d
- **Results:**
  - 10 MMR-deficient colorectal cancers
    - Immune-related ORR: 40% and immune-related PFS: 78%
    - Median PFS and OS not reached
  - 18 MMR-proficient colorectal cancers
    - Immune-related ORR: 0% and immune-related PFS: 11%
    - Median PFS: 2 months
    - Median OS: 5 months

- Seven MMR-deficient non-colorectal cancers
  - Immune-related ORR: 71% and immune-related PFS: 67%
  - Cohort C included two endometrial cancer patients, one with PR and one with CR
- MMR-deficient cancers with mean of 1,782 mutations per tumor vs. 73 in MMR-proficient cancers
  - High somatic mutation load associated with prolonged PFS
- **Conclusion:**
  - → MMR status predicts clinical benefit of immune checkpoint blockade with pembrolizumab

Study: Keynote-158

- **Citation:** (Marabelle et al., 2020)
- **Highlight:** Pembrolizumab in MSI-H/ dMMR solid tumors, including endometrial cancer
- **Background:** Genomes of tumor with deficient DNA mismatch repair (dMMR) have high microsatellite instability (MSI-H) and many somatic mutations that encode potential neoantigens
- **Design:**
  - Phase II study: 233 patients with MSI-H/dMMR non-colorectal cancers ≥1 prior therapy received pembrolizumab iv 200 mg q 3 weeks
- **Results:**
  - 27 tumor types, most common endometrial, gastric, cholangiocarcinoma, and pancreatic cancer
  - ORR: 34.3%
  - Median PFS: 4.1 months
  - Median OS: 23.5 months
  - ≥Grade 3 AEs in 14.6%
  - 49/233 with endometrial cancer
    - ORR: 57.1%
    - Median PFS: 25.7 months
    - Median OS: Not reached
    - Median DOR: Not reached
- **Conclusion:**
  - → Clinical benefit of pembrolizumab with unresectable or metastatic MSI-H/ dMMR non-colorectal cancer

Study: Keynote-028

- **Citation:** (Ott et al., 2017)
- **Highlight:** Pembrolizumab in PD-L1-positive endometrial cancer
- **Design:**
  - Multicohort phase IB study, presented here results of endometrial cancer cohort: 24 patients with advanced PD-L1-positive endometrial cancer and progression after standard therapy received pembrolizumab
  - 10 mg/kg pembrolizumab q 2 weeks

- **Results:**
  - 15/24 received at least two prior lines
  - PR: 3 /24 (13%); median DOR not reached
  - SD: 3/24 (13%); median duration of 24.6 weeks
  - Grade 3 AEs in 4/24 patients; no grade 4
- **Conclusion:**
  - → Pembrolizumab with favorable safety profile and durable antitumor activity in heavily pretreated advanced PD-L1-positive endometrial cancer

Study: GARNET

- **Citation:** (Oaknin et al., 2020)
- **Highlight:** TSR-042, humanized monoclonal PD-1 antibody
- **Design:**
  - Phase I multicohort trial: 71 patients with PD-L1 + advanced or recurrent pretreated, microsatellite instability-high (MSI-H) or mismatch repair deficient (dMMR) endometrial cancer received anti-PD-L1 monoclonal antibody, TSR-042, 500 mg q 3 wks for four doses, then 1,000 mg q 6 wks
- **Results:**
  - Median follow-up: 11.2 months
  - CR: 9/71 (12.7%)
  - PR: 30/71 (42.3%)
  - SD: 11/71 (15.5%)
  - PD: 27/71 (38%)
  - Mean DOR: Not reached
    - Estimated likelihood of maintaining response: 76.8% at 12 months
  - ≥Grade 3 AE: Anemia (2.9%), colitis (1.9%), and diarrhea (1.9%)
- **Conclusion:**
  - → Robust clinical activity and acceptable toxicity

Study: Keynote-146/Study 111

- **Citation:** (Makker et al., 2020)
- **Highlight:** Lenvatinib plus pembrolizumab in advanced endometrial cancer
- **Background:**
  - Lenvatinib = multi-kinase inhibitor of VEGFR1–3 and other tyrosine kinases
- **Design:**
  - Phase Ib/II trial of 108 patients with advanced endometrial cancer, unselected for microsatellite instability or PD-L1 untreated or with ≤2 prior lines received 20 mg lenvatinib po qd plus 200 mg pembrolizumab iv q 3 wks
- **Results:**
  - Median follow-up: 18.7 months
  - Uterine serous carcinoma in 32.4%

- PD-L1 status
  - Positive: 49.1%
  - Negative: 39.8%
  - Unknown: 11.1%
- Microsatellite status
  - MSI-H: 10.2%
  - MSS: 87%
- ORR at 24 wks: 38%
  - ORR at 24 wks in MSI-H: 89.1%
  - ORR at 24 wks in MS-S: 36.2%
- For previously treated patients
  - Median DOR: 21.2 months
  - Median PFS: 7.4 months
  - Median OS: 16.7 months
- Grade ≥3 AEs in 66.9%
- Dose reductions of lenvatinib in 62.9%
- Mean dose intensity of lenvatinib: 14.4 mg/d
- **Conclusion:**
  - → Lenvatinib plus pembrolizumab with antitumor activity in advanced endometrial cancer who experienced disease progression after prior systemic therapy, regardless of MSI status
  - Manageable toxicity profile

Study: Study 309/Keynote-775

- **Citation:** (Makker et al., 2022)
- **Highlight:** Lenvatinib plus pembrolizumab in advanced endometrial cancer
- **Design:**
  - 827 patients with measurable advanced, recurrent endometrial cancers, 697 pMMR (proficient MMR) and 103 dMMR, with progression of disease after one previous platinum-based CT, randomized to 20 mg lenvatinib po qd plus 200 mg pembrolizumab iv q 3 wks vs. 60 mg/m^2 doxorubicin q 4 weeks or weekly 80 mg/m^2 paclitaxel
- **Results:**
  - 25.1% uterine serous carcinoma in lenvima + pembro group
  - Median PFS
    - pMMR: 6.6 vs. 3.8 months (HR 0.6; CI = 0.5–0.72; $p < 0.001$) (lenvima + pembro vs. CT)
    - Overall: 7.2 vs. 3.8 months
  - Median OS
    - pMMR: 17.4 vs. 12.0 months (HR 0.68; CI = 0.56–0.84; $p < 0.001$)
    - Overall: 18.3 vs. 11.4 months
  - Grade ≥3 AEs: 88.9% vs. 72.7%
    - Most common in lenvima + pembro group hypertension
    - In 66.5% dose reduction of lenvatinib

- **Conclusion:**
  - → Lenvatinib plus pembrolizumab led to significantly longer PFS and OS than CT in advanced endometrial cancer

1.2 UTERINE CARCINOSARCOMA

1.2.1 Studies Addressing Prognosticators

Study: GOG 40

- **Citation:** (Major et al., 1993)
- **Highlight:** Sites of recurrence and prognostic factors for mixed mesodermal tumors (MMTs) and leiomyosarcomas (LMS)
- **Design:**
  - Retrospective cohort study of clinical stage I and II uterine sarcoma
  - 453 patients evaluable and analyzed for prognostic factors
- **Results:**
  - 301 MMT (167 homologous; 134 heterologous); 59 LMS; remaining 93 sarcomas mainly stromal cell and adenosarcomas
  - Here, only MMT and LMS analyzed
  - Recurrence rate of MMT: 53%
    - Site of first recurrence: 21% pelvis (only 9.3% in lungs)
  - Recurrence rate of LMS: 71%
    - Site of first recurrence: 14% pelvis (40.7% in lungs)
  - Prognostic factors for MMT in multivariate analysis
    - Adnexal spread, LN metastasis, histologic cell type (homologous vs. heterologous), and grade of sarcoma
  - Prognostic factors for LMS in multivariate analysis
    - Mitotic index

1.2.2 Studies Addressing Adjuvant Treatment

Study: GOG 117

- **Citation:** (Sutton et al., 2005)
- **Highlight:** Ifosfamide/ mesna + cisplatin
- **Design:**
  - Phase II trial: 65 patients with completely resected stage I or II carcinosarcoma and no postoperative RT received adjuvant ifosfamide/ mesna and cisplatin

- Ifosfamide 1.5 g/m^2 over 1 h and cisplatin 20 mg/m^2 over 15 min followed by mesna 120 mg/m^2 iv bolus, then 1.5 mg/m^2/24 h continuous infusion qd × 5 d q 3 wks × 3 C
- **Results:**
  - Initial doses were dose reduced by 20% for myelotoxicity (i.e., continuous infusion instead of 5 d only 4 d)
  - 2-yr PFS: 69%
    - \>50% of recurrences involved pelvis and vagina
  - 2-yr OS: 82%
  - 5-yr OS: 62%
  - Leukopenia most common toxicity
- **Conclusion:**
  - → Adjuvant ifosfamide and cisplatin for stage I/II carcinosarcoma is tolerable regimen
  - No controls, therefore, impact on PFS and OS unclear; pelvic recurrence remains problematic

Study: GOG 150

- **Citation:** (Wolfson et al., 2007)
- **Highlight:** Whole abdominal irradiation (WAI)
- **Design:**
  - Based on GOG 20 and GOG 40
  - 206 patients with stage I–IV carcinosarcoma after optimal cytoreductive surgery and no extra-abdominal disease randomized to WAI (30 Gy to whole abdomen using EBRT followed by pelvic boost to cumulative pelvic dose of 50 Gy) vs. 3 C cisplatin–ifosfamide and mesna (CIM) (cisplatin 20 mg/m^2 qd × 4 d; ifosfamide 1.5 g/m^2 qd × 4 d; mesna 120 mg/m^2 iv bolus over 15 min on day 1 followed by 1.5 g/m^2 qd continuous infusion × 4 d)
- **Results:**
  - Stage I 31%, stage II 13%, stage III 45%, and stage IV 12%
  - 5-yr recurrence rate: 58% vs. 52% (WAI vs. CIM)
    - Sites of recurrence:
      - Vagina: 4/105 vs. 10/101
      - Pelvis: 14 vs. 14
      - Abdomen: 29 vs. 19
      - Lung: 14 vs. 14
      - Other distant: 13 vs. 10
  - Adjusted for stage and age, recurrence rate 21% lower for CIM but not significant (p = 0.245)
  - Estimated death rate 29% lower for CIM but not significant (p = 0.085)
  - More late toxicities in WAI, mainly GI (p < 0.001), including two patients died of radiation-induced hepatitis
- **Conclusion:**
  - → No statistically significant advantage in recurrence rate or survival, but trend favors CT

1.2.3 Studies Addressing Treatment of Advanced/Recurrent Uterine Carcinosarcoma

Study: GOG 108

- **Citation:** (Sutton et al., 2000)
- **Highlight:** Ifosfamide/ mesna +/– cisplatin
- **Design:**
  - 194 patients with advanced, persistent, or recurrent carcinosarcoma without prior CT randomized to ifosfamide 1.5 g/m^2/d ($\times$ 5 d q 3 wks) plus mesna vs. ifosfamide/ mesna and cisplatin 10 mg/m^2/d ($\times$ 5 d)
- **Results:**
  - Early in study, 20% dose reduction for combination therapy because of toxicity
    - Grade 3 or 4 granulocytopenia: 36% vs. 60% (single vs. combination)
    - Grade 3 or anemia: 8% vs. 17%
    - Grade 3 or 4 CNS toxicity: 19% vs. 14%
    - Grade 3 or 4 peripheral neuropathy: 1% vs. 12%
    - Treatment may have contributed to the death of six patients treated with full dose of ifosfamide and cisplatin
  - ORR: 36% vs. 54%; pelvic: 47% vs. 61%; lung: 21% vs. 54%: other metastatic sites: 33% vs. 40% (single vs. combination); OR 1.82 (p = 0.03)
  - PFS RR: 0.73 for combination (upper confidence limit 0.94; p = 0.02)
  - OS RR: 0.8 (upper limit 1.03; p = 0.071)
- **Conclusion:**
  - → Addition of cisplatin with small improvement in PFS but no survival benefit; however, added toxicity may not justify use of combination

Study: GOG 161

- **Citation:** (Homesley et al., 2007)
- **Highlight:** Ifosfamide/ mesna +/– paclitaxel
- **Design:**
  - 179 patients with measurable stage III or IV, persistent or recurrent carcinosarcoma randomized to ifosfamide (2.0 mg/m^2 qd $\times$ 3 d) plus mesna q 3 wks vs. ifosfamide (1.6 mg/m^2 qd $\times$ 3 d) plus mesna and paclitaxel (135 mg/m^2 over 3 hrs) plus filgrastim (started on day 4) q 3 wks
- **Results:**
  - Sensory neuropathy grade 1–4: 8% vs. 30% (single vs. combination)
  - ORR: 29% vs. 45%
  - PFS: 3.6 vs. 5.8 months; 29% decrease in HR (p = 0.03)
  - OS: 8.4 vs. 13.5 months; 31% decrease in HR (p = 0.03)
- **Conclusion:**
  - → OS significantly improved; toxicities manageable

Study: GOG 232B

- **Citation:** (Powell et al., 2010)
- **Highlight:** Carboplatin + paclitaxel
- **Background:**
  - Platinum and taxane compounds showed activity in uterine carcinosarcoma (uCS); ifosfamide plus paclitaxel established superiority to ifosfamide alone based on phase III trial; however, toxicity and multiday schedule → further development of novel regimens needed
- **Design:**
  - Phase II trial: 46 patients with measurable stage III or IV, persistent or recurrent carcinosarcoma, and no prior CT received paclitaxel (175 mg/m^2 over 3 hrs) and carboplatin (AUC 6) q 3 wks until progression or toxicity
- **Results:**
  - 59% completed 6 C or more
  - ORR: 54% (CR 13%; PR 41%)
- **Conclusion:**
  - → Combination with activity and acceptable toxicity

Study: GOG 261

- **Citation:** (Powell et al., 2022)
- **Design:**
  - In non-inferiority trial, 449 patients with newly diagnosed or recurrent uCS and 90 with ovarian carcinosarcoma randomized to paclitaxel 175 mg/m^2 plus carboplatin AUC 6 vs. 1.6 g/m^2 ifosfamide on days 1–3 and mesna plus paclitaxel 135 mg/m^2 on day 1
- **Results:**
  - Uterine carcinosarcoma
    - Median PFS: 16 vs. 12 months (Taxol + carbo vs. ifos + Taxol)
    - Median OS: 37 vs. 29 months
  - Ovarian carcinosarcoma
    - Median PFS: 15 vs. 10 months
    - Median OS: 30 vs. 25 months
  - No new safety signals with either regimen
- **Conclusion:**
  - → Paclitaxel plus carboplatin was not inferior to ifosfamide plus paclitaxel and should be standard of treatment for uCS

Study: ROCSAN trial

- **Citation:** NCT03651206; ongoing (Ray-Coquard et al., 2021)
- **Background:** Gynecological carcinosarcomas (CS) rare and highly aggressive with a 5-yr OS <10%; median PFS after platinum-based CT <4 months and median OS <1 yr

- **Design:**
  - Phase II: 63 patients with recurrent or progressive endometrial or ovarian CS after at least first-line platinum-based CT randomized 2:2:1 to receive niraparib vs. niraparib + dostarlimab vs. standard CT (paclitaxel, doxorubicin, gemcitabine, or topotecan)
  - Stratification by number of prior lines, stage, CS localization, and performance status

1.3 UTERINE LEIOMYOSARCOMA

1.3.1 Studies Addressing Adjuvant Treatment of Early-Stage Uterine Leiomyosarcoma

Study: GOG 20

- **Citation:** (Omura et al., 1985)
- **Highlight:** Doxorubicin vs. observation
- **Background:**
  - Doxorubicin had been used alone or in various combinations in palliative treatment of metastatic soft-tissue sarcomas and appeared highly effective; therefore, doxorubicin in GOG 20 used in adjuvant setting
- **Design:**
  - 156 patients with stage I and II uterine sarcomas after surgery and optional postoperative radiation (external or intracavitary) randomized to adjuvant treatment with doxorubicin (Adriamycin®) for 6 months vs. observation
- **Results:**
  - No difference in recurrences in 31/75 vs. 43/81 (doxorubicin vs. observation)
  - No difference in PFS or OS
  - Optional RT did not influence outcome; suggestion that vaginal recurrences decreased by pelvic RT
  - Recurrence rate in specific cell types not significantly different, but pattern of recurrence differed
    - Pulmonary mets more common in LMS
    - Extrapulmonary/pelvic mets more common in carcinosarcoma
- **Conclusion:**
  - → No benefit of adjuvant doxorubicin

Study: EORTEC 55874

- **Citation:** (Reed et al., 2008)
- **Highlight:** Pelvic RT vs. observation for uterine sarcomas

- **Design:**
  - 1987–2000: 224 patients with stage I and II uterine sarcomas s/p at minimum hysterectomy/BSO/washings (nodal sampling optional) randomized to pelvic radiation (51 Gy in 28 fractions over 5 wks) vs. observation
- **Results:**
  - 103 LMS, 91 CS, and 28 endometrial stromal sarcomas (ESSs)
  - Overall
    - Local recurrences: 14 vs. 24 (p = 0.004) (RT vs. observation)
    - No effect on PFS or OS
  - Increased local control for CS but not for LMS
- **Conclusion:**
  - No benefit from pelvic RT for LMS

Study: SARC 005

- **Citation:** (Hensley et al., 2013)
- **Highlight:** Gemcitabine/docetaxel + doxorubicin
- **Background:**
  - 30–50% with high-grade uterine leiomyosarcoma (uLMS) limited to uterus at diagnosis remain progression-free at 2 yrs; pelvic RT does not improve outcomes
- **Design:**
  - Phase II trial: 46 patients with high-grade uLMS limited to the uterus after surgery received adjuvant 4 C of gemcitabine–docetaxel; if disease-free on CT after 4 C received 4 C of doxorubicin
- **Results:**
  - Stage I 81%; stage II 15%; serosa-only stage IIIA 4%
  - Median tumor size: 8 cm (2.5–30 cm)
  - Median mitotic rate: 18 mitoses per 10 HPF
  - 89% received all planned 8 C of adjuvant CT
  - At median follow-up time of 39.8 months, 21/46 (45.7%) developed recurrence; median PFS was not reached
  - Median time to recurrence: 27.4 months (range: 3–40 months)
  - 2-yr PFS: 78%; 3-yr PFS: 57%
- **Conclusion:**
  - → In high-grade uterus-limited uLMS who received adjuvant gemcitabine plus docetaxel followed by doxorubicin, 2-yr PFS 78%

Study: GOG 277

- **Citation:** (Hensley et al., 2018)
- **Highlight:** Gemcitabine/docetaxel plus doxorubicin vs. observation in uterine confined uLMS
- **Design:**
  - Phase III trial: Patients with stage I high-risk uLMS confined to uterus +/– cervix imaging confirmed disease-free s/p hysterectomy randomized to gemcitabine and docetaxel followed by doxorubicin vs. observation

- 4 C gemcitabine–docetaxel and if disease-free on CT + MRI, 4 additional C doxorubicin
- Gemcitabine 900 mg/m^2 over 90 min on days 1 and 8, docetaxel 75 mg/m^2 on day 8, GCSF 5 µg/kg on days 9–15 or pegfilgrastim 6 mg on day 9 or 10, plus doxorubicin 60 mg/m^2 q 21 d
- June 2012–September 2016, at 701 international sites; target accrual 216
- **Results:**
  - Actual accrual 38, closed per NCI early stopping guidelines for poor accrual
  - 20 assigned to CT; 18 to observation
    - 3/20 never received CT
  - ≥Grade 3 AEs: 47% vs. <1% (CT vs. observation)
  - 4-yr restricted mean OS: 34.3 vs. 46.4 months
  - 2-yr restricted mean RFS: 18.1 vs. 14.6 months
- **Conclusion:**
  - Despite international collaboration, study closed due to poor accrual
  - Data do not suggest survival benefit to multi-agent adjuvant CT
  - Observation following complete intact resection of uterus-limited uLMS remains standard of care

1.3.2 Studies Addressing Treatment of Advanced Uterine Leiomyosarcoma

Study: Hensley study

- **Citation:** (Hensley et al., 2002)
- **Highlight:** Gemcitabine + docetaxel
- **Design:**
  - Phase II trial: 34 patients with unresectable LMS not responding to zero to two prior chemotherapies (particularly progressed after doxorubicin) received gemcitabine (900 mg/m^2 on days 1 and 8) and docetaxel (100 mg/m^2 on day 8) with G-CSF given on days 9–15
  - If prior pelvic RT, 25% lower dose
  - Gemcitabine delivered over 30 or 90 min in C 1 and 2 and by 90 min infusion in all subsequent cycles
- **Results:**
  - Pharmacokinetics
    - Every patient is own control: if in C1 infusion over 30 min, then in C2 over 90 min and vice versa
    - Duration of gemcitabine concentration remained above 10 µmol/L 50% longer with 90 min infusion compared with 30 min infusion
    - However, trend to lower peak concentrations with 90 min infusion
  - 18/34 patients without prior CT
  - 16/34 had progressed after doxorubicin-based therapy
  - Hematologic toxicity common, but neutropenic fever or bleeding rare

- – Neutropenia: Grade 3 in 15%; grade 4 in 6%
- – Thrombocytopenia: Grade 3 in 26%; grade 4 in 3%
- – Neutropenic fever: 6%
- – Bleeding: 0%
- ORR: 53% (CR 3/34; PR 15/34)
- 50% of responders previously treated with doxorubicin
- SD in seven patients
- PFS: 5.6 months
- **Conclusion:**
  - → Combination of gemcitabine/docetaxel tolerable and highly active in treated and untreated LMS

Study: GOG 131G

- **Citation:** (Hensley et al., 2008a)
- **Highlight:** Gemcitabine + docetaxel (second line)
- **Design:**
  - Phase II trial: 48 patients with unresectable metastatic uLMS progressing after prior CT received as second-line treatment gemcitabine (900 mg/m^2 over 90 min on days 1 and 8) and docetaxel 100 mg/m^2 on day 8 and GCSF days 9–21
- **Background:**
  - Use of fixed-dose rate infusion of gemcitabine: To maintain gemcitabine concentration at a level that optimizes incorporation of active gemcitabine metabolite (gemcitabine triphosphate) into DNA (gemcitabine = nucleoside analog, imitates cytidine, 'faulty base'); preferred over bolus infusion
    - – Doxorubicin was first line for metastatic uLMS with 25% response rate
    - – Combination doxorubicin with ifosfamide did not show improved outcome
    - – Ifosfamide alone, response rate: 17.2%
    - – Gemcitabine alone, response rate: 20%
- **Results:**
  - Prior therapy in 90% doxorubicin-based and in 6% ifosfamide-based
  - Patients with prior pelvic RT received lower doses
  - Main toxicity: Uncomplicated myelosuppression
    - – Thrombocytopenia grade 3 in 29%, grade 4 in 10.4%; neutropenia grade 3 in 12.5%, grade 4 in 8.3%; anemia grade 3 in 20.8%, grade 4 in 4.2%
    - – Pulmonary toxicity reported, but no patient with drug-related pneumonitis/ hypoxia-type toxicity
  - Median number of cycles received: 5.5
  - ORR: 27% (CR 6.3%; PR 20.8%)
  - SD: 50% (median duration: 5.4 months)
  - Median PFS: 5.6 months
  - Median DOR: 9 months

- **Conclusion:**
  - → Fixed-dose rate gemcitabine and docetaxel is active second-line treatment for metastatic uLMS (first line: doxorubicin-based)

Study: GOG 87L

- **Citation:** (Hensley et al., 2008b)
- **Highlight:** Gemcitabine + docetaxel (first line)
- **Design:**
  - Phase II trial: 39 patients with metastatic uLMS received as first-line treatment gemcitabine (900 mg/m^2 over 90 min on days 1 and 8) and docetaxel 100 mg/m^2 on day 8 and GCSF days 9–21 as until progression or toxicity
- **Results:**
  - 50% received 6 or more C
  - Myelosuppression
  - ORR: 35.8% (CR 4.8%; PR 31%)
  - Median DOR: 6 months
  - SD: 26.2%
  - Median PFS: 4.4 months
  - Median OS: 16+ months (range: 4–41.3 months)
- **Conclusion:**
  - → Gemcitabine + docetaxel achieved high objective response rate as first-line therapy in metastatic uLMS

Study: GOG 231C

- **Citation:** (Hensley et al., 2009)
- **Highlight:** Sunitinib
- **Design:**
  - Phase II trial: 23 patients with recurrent or persistent uLMS after one to two prior chemotherapies received sunitinib malate (50 mg po qd × 4 wks), then 2 wks rest; assessment after 6 wks
  - Sunitinib = Receptor tyrosine kinase inhibitor, including PDGF-R and VEGFR
- **Results:**
  - PR: 2/23
  - SD at 6 months: 4/23
  - PFS: 1.5 months
- **Conclusion:**
  - → Sunitinib fails to achieve objective response or SD

Study: Hensley study

- **Citation:** (Hensley et al., 2015)
- **Highlight:** Gemcitabine/docetaxel +/– BEV

- **Background:**
  - Fixed-dose rate gemcitabine plus docetaxel with objective response of 35% (GOG 87L); determine if addition of BEV is beneficial
- **Design:**
  - Phase III trial: 107 patients with metastatic unresectable uLMS without prior CT randomized to gemcitabine, docetaxel, and BEV vs. gemcitabine, docetaxel, and placebo
- **Results:**
  - Accrual stopped early for futility; planned target accrual was 130 to resolve difference in median PFS from 4 and 6.7 months
  - No difference in grade 3 and 4 toxicities
  - ORR: 31.5% vs. 35.8%; mean duration of response 8.6 vs. 8.8 months (gemcitabine–docetaxel vs. gemcitabine-docetaxel plus BEV)
  - PFS: 6.2 vs. 4.2 months
  - OS: 26.9 vs. 23.3 months
- **Conclusion:**
  - → Addition of BEV to first-line treatment of metastatic uLMS failed to improve PFS, OS, and ORR; gemcitabine–docetaxel remains first-line treatment for uLMS

Study: GeDDiS trial (Gemcitabine et Docetaxel vs. Doxorubicin in Sarcoma)

- **Citation:** (Seddon et al., 2017)
- **Highlight:** Gemcitabine and docetaxel vs. doxorubicin
- **Design:**
  - 257 patients with locally advanced or metastatic soft-tissue grade 2 or 3 sarcoma randomized to doxorubicin 75 mg/m^2 on day 1 q 3 wks vs. gemcitabine 675 mg/m^2 on days 1 and 8 and docetaxel 75 mg/m^2 on day 1 q 3 weeks
  - Randomization stratified by age and histological subtype
    - uLMS: 28% vs. 27%
    - Non-uterine LMS: 19% vs. 18%
    - Synovial sarcoma: 4% vs. 5%
    - Pleomorphic sarcoma: 12% vs. 13%
    - Other: 56% vs. 55%
- **Results:**
  - Median follow-up: 22 months
  - Proportion alive and progression free: 46.3% vs. 46.4% (doxorubicin vs. gemcitabine/docetaxel)
  - PFS: 23.3 vs. 23.7 wks (HR 1.28; CI: 0.99–1.65; p = 0.06)
    - CR: 2% vs. 0%
    - PR: 18% vs. 20%
    - SD: 47% vs. 39%
    - PD: 19% vs. 21%
  - ≥Grade 3 AE:
    - Neutropenia: 25% vs. 20%

- Febrile neutropenia: 20% vs. 12%
- Fatigue: 6% vs. 14%
- Oral mucositis: 14% vs. 2%
- Pain: 8% vs. 10%

- **Conclusion:**
  - → Doxorubicin should remain standard first line for most patients with advanced soft-tissue sarcoma

REFERENCES

Aghajanian, C., Filiaci, V., Dizon, D.S., Carlson, J.W., Powell, M.A., Secord, A.A., Tewari, K.S., Bender, D.P., O'Malley, D.M., Stuckey, A., et al. (2018). A phase II study of frontline paclitaxel/carboplatin/bevacizumab, paclitaxel/carboplatin/temsirolimus, or ixabepilone/carboplatin/bevacizumab in advanced/recurrent endometrial cancer. Gynecol Oncol *150*, 274–281. 10.1016/j.ygyno.2018.05.018.

Aghajanian, C., Sill, M.W., Darcy, K.M., Greer, B., McMeekin, D.S., Rose, P.G., Rotmensch, J., Barnes, M.N., Hanjani, P., and Leslie, K.K. (2011). Phase II trial of bevacizumab in recurrent or persistent endometrial cancer: a Gynecologic Oncology Group study. J Clin Oncol *29*, 2259–2265. 10.1200/JCO.2010.32.6397.

Alvarez, E.A., Brady, W.E., Walker, J.L., Rotmensch, J., Zhou, X.C., Kendrick, J.E., Yamada, S.D., Schilder, J.M., Cohn, D.E., Harrison, C.R., et al. (2013). Phase II trial of combination bevacizumab and temsirolimus in the treatment of recurrent or persistent endometrial carcinoma: a Gynecologic Oncology Group study. Gynecol Oncol *129*, 22–27. 10.1016/j.ygyno.2012.12.022.

ASTEC/EN.5 Study Group, Blake, P., Swart, A.M., Orton, J., Kitchener, H., Whelan, T., Lukka, H., Eisenhauer, E., Bacon, M., Tu, D., et al. (2009a). Adjuvant external beam radiotherapy in the treatment of endometrial cancer (MRC ASTEC and NCIC CTG EN.5 randomised trials): pooled trial results, systematic review, and meta-analysis. Lancet *373*, 137–146. 10.1016/S0140-6736(08)61767-5.

ASTEC Study Group, Kitchener, H., Swart, A.M., Qian, Q., Amos, C., and Parmar, M.K. (2009b). Efficacy of systematic pelvic lymphadenectomy in endometrial cancer (MRC ASTEC trial): a randomised study. Lancet *373*, 125–136. 10.1016/S0140-6736(08)61766-3.

Ballester, M., Dubernard, G., Lecuru, F., Heitz, D., Mathevet, P., Marret, H., Querleu, D., Golfier, F., Leblanc, E., Rouzier, R., and Darai, E. (2011). Detection rate and diagnostic accuracy of sentinel-node biopsy in early stage endometrial cancer: a prospective multicentre study (SENTI-ENDO). Lancet Oncol *12*, 469–476. 10.1016/S1470-2045(11)70070-5.

Benedetti Panici, P., Basile, S., Maneschi, F., Alberto Lissoni, A., Signorelli, M., Scambia, G., Angioli, R., Tateo, S., Mangili, G., Katsaros, D., et al. (2008). Systematic pelvic lymphadenectomy vs. no lymphadenectomy in early-stage endometrial carcinoma: randomized clinical trial. J Natl Cancer Inst *100*, 1707–1716. 10.1093/jnci/djn397.

Creasman, W.T., Morrow, C.P., Bundy, B.N., Homesley, H.D., Graham, J.E., and Heller, P.B. (1987). Surgical pathologic spread patterns of endometrial cancer. a Gynecologic Oncology Group study. Cancer *60*, 2035–2041.

Creutzberg, C.L., Nout, R.A., Lybeert, M.L., Warlam-Rodenhuis, C.C., Jobsen, J.J., Mens, J.W., Lutgens, L.C., Pras, E., van de Poll-Franse, L.V., van Putten, W.L., and Group, P.S. (2011).

Fifteen-year radiotherapy outcomes of the randomized PORTEC-1 trial for endometrial carcinoma. Int J Radiat Oncol Biol Phys *81*, e631–e638. 10.1016/j.ijrobp.2011.04.013.

Creutzberg, C.L., van Putten, W.L., Koper, P.C., Lybeert, M.L., Jobsen, J.J., Warlam-Rodenhuis, C.C., De Winter, K.A., Lutgens, L.C., van den Bergh, A.C., van de Steen-Banasik, E., et al. (2000). Surgery and postoperative radiotherapy versus surgery alone for patients with stage-1 endometrial carcinoma: multicentre randomised trial. PORTEC Study Group. Post Operative Radiation Therapy in Endometrial Carcinoma. Lancet *355*, 1404–1411.

Cusimano, M.C., Vicus, D., Pulman, K., Maganti, M., Bernardini, M.Q., Bouchard-Fortier, G., Laframboise, S., May, T., Hogen, L.F., Covens, A.L., et al. (2021). Assessment of Sentinel Lymph Node Biopsy vs Lymphadenectomy for Intermediate- and High-Grade Endometrial Cancer Staging. JAMA Surg *156*, 157–164. 10.1001/jamasurg.2020.5060.

de Boer, S.M., Powell, M.E., Mileshkin, L., Katsaros, D., Bessette, P., Haie-Meder, C., Ottevanger, P.B., Ledermann, J.A., Khaw, P., Colombo, A., et al. (2016). Toxicity and quality of life after adjuvant chemoradiotherapy versus radiotherapy alone for women with high-risk endometrial cancer (PORTEC-3): an open-label, multicentre, randomised, phase 3 trial. Lancet Oncol *17*, 1114–1126. 10.1016/S1470–2045(16)30120-6.

de Boer, S.M., Powell, M.E., Mileshkin, L., Katsaros, D., Bessette, P., Haie-Meder, C., Ottevanger, P.B., Ledermann, J.A., Khaw, P., Colombo, A., et al. (2018). Adjuvant chemoradiotherapy versus radiotherapy alone for women with high-risk endometrial cancer (PORTEC-3): final results of an international, open-label, multicentre, randomised, phase 3 trial. Lancet Oncol *19*, 295–309. 10.1016/S1470-2045(18)30079-2.

Fader, A.N., Roque, D.M., Siegel, E., Buza, N., Hui, P., Abdelghany, O., Chambers, S.K., Secord, A.A., Havrilesky, L., O'Malley, D.M., et al. (2018). Randomized phase II trial of carboplatin-paclitaxel versus carboplatin-paclitaxel-trastuzumab in uterine serous carcinomas that overexpress human epidermal growth factor receptor 2/neu. J Clin Oncol *36*, 2044–2051. 10.1200/JCO.2017.76.5966.

Fiorica, J.V., Brunetto, V.L., Hanjani, P., Lentz, S.S., Mannel, R., Andersen, W., and Gynecologic Oncology Group, S. (2004). Phase II trial of alternating courses of megestrol acetate and tamoxifen in advanced endometrial carcinoma: a Gynecologic Oncology Group study. Gynecol Oncol *92*, 10–14.

Fleming, G.F., Brunetto, V.L., Cella, D., Look, K.Y., Reid, G.C., Munkarah, A.R., Kline, R., Burger, R.A., Goodman, A., and Burks, R.T. (2004a). Phase III trial of doxorubicin plus cisplatin with or without paclitaxel plus filgrastim in advanced endometrial carcinoma: a Gynecologic Oncology Group study. J Clin Oncol *22*, 2159–2166. 10.1200/JCO.2004.07.184.

Fleming, G.F., Filiaci, V.L., Bentley, R.C., Herzog, T., Sorosky, J., Vaccarello, L., and Gallion, H. (2004b). Phase III randomized trial of doxorubicin + cisplatin versus doxorubicin + 24-h paclitaxel + filgrastim in endometrial carcinoma: a Gynecologic Oncology Group study. Ann Oncol *15*, 1173–1178. 10.1093/annonc/mdh316.

Fleming, G.F., Filiaci, V.L., Marzullo, B., Zaino, R.J., Davidson, S.A., Pearl, M., Makker, V., Burke, J.J., 2nd, Zweizig, S.L., Van Le, L., et al. (2014c). Temsirolimus with or without megestrol acetate and tamoxifen for endometrial cancer: a Gynecologic Oncology Group study. Gynecol Oncol *132*, 585–592. 10.1016/j.ygyno.2014.01.015.

Fleming, N.D., Coleman, R.L., Tung, C., Westin, S.N., Hu, W., Sun, Y., Bhosale, P., Munsell, M.F., and Sood, A.K. (2017). Phase II trial of bevacizumab with dose-dense paclitaxel as first-line treatment in patients with advanced ovarian cancer. Gynecol Oncol *147*, 41–46. 10.1016/j.ygyno.2017.07.137.

Greven, K., Winter, K., Underhill, K., Fontenesci, J., Cooper, J., and Burke, T. (2006). Final analysis of RTOG 9708: adjuvant postoperative irradiation combined with cisplatin/paclitaxel chemotherapy following surgery for patients with high-risk endometrial cancer. Gynecol Oncol *103*, 155–159. 10.1016/j.ygyno.2006.02.007.

Greven, K., Winter, K., Underhill, K., Fontenesci, J., Cooper, J., Burke, T., and Radiation Therapy Oncology, G. (2004). Preliminary analysis of RTOG 9708: adjuvant postoperative radiotherapy combined with cisplatin/paclitaxel chemotherapy after surgery for patients with high-risk endometrial cancer. Int J Radiat Oncol Biol Phys *59*, 168–173. 10.1016/j.ijrobp.2003.10.019.

Hensley, M.L., Blessing, J.A., Degeest, K., Abulafia, O., Rose, P.G., and Homesley, H.D. (2008a). Fixed-dose rate gemcitabine plus docetaxel as second-line therapy for metastatic uterine leiomyosarcoma: a Gynecologic Oncology Group phase II study. Gynecol Oncol *109*, 323–328. 10.1016/j.ygyno.2008.02.024.

Hensley, M.L., Blessing, J.A., Mannel, R., and Rose, P.G. (2008b). Fixed-dose rate gemcitabine plus docetaxel as first-line therapy for metastatic uterine leiomyosarcoma: a Gynecologic Oncology Group phase II trial. Gynecol Oncol *109*, 329–334. 10.1016/j.ygyno.2008.03.010.

Hensley, M.L., Enserro, D., Hatcher, H., Ottevanger, P.B., Krarup-Hansen, A., Blay, J.Y., Fisher, C., Moxley, K.M., Lele, S.B., Lea, J.S., et al. (2018). Adjuvant gemcitabine plus docetaxel followed by doxorubicin versus observation for high-grade uterine leiomyosarcoma: a phase III NRG oncology/Gynecologic Oncology Group study. J Clin Oncol, JCO1800454. 10.1200/JCO.18.00454.

Hensley, M.L., Maki, R., Venkatraman, E., Geller, G., Lovegren, M., Aghajanian, C., Sabbatini, P., Tong, W., Barakat, R., and Spriggs, D.R. (2002). Gemcitabine and docetaxel in patients with unresectable leiomyosarcoma: results of a phase II trial. J Clin Oncol *20*, 2824–2831. 10.1200/JCO.2002.11.050.

Hensley, M.L., Miller, A., O'Malley, D.M., Mannel, R.S., Behbakht, K., Bakkum-Gamez, J.N., and Michael, H. (2015). Randomized phase III trial of gemcitabine plus docetaxel plus bevacizumab or placebo as first-line treatment for metastatic uterine leiomyosarcoma: an NRG oncology/Gynecologic Oncology Group study. J Clin Oncol *33*, 1180–1185. 10.1200/JCO.2014.58.3781.

Hensley, M.L., Sill, M.W., Scribner, D.R., Jr., Brown, J., Debernardo, R.L., Hartenbach, E.M., McCourt, C.K., Bosscher, J.R., and Gehrig, P.A. (2009). Sunitinib malate in the treatment of recurrent or persistent uterine leiomyosarcoma: a Gynecologic Oncology Group phase II study. Gynecol Oncol *115*, 460–465. 10.1016/j.ygyno.2009.09.011.

Hensley, M.L., Wathen, J.K., Maki, R.G., Araujo, D.M., Sutton, G., Priebat, D.A., George, S., Soslow, R.A., and Baker, L.H. (2013). Adjuvant therapy for high-grade, uterus-limited leiomyosarcoma: results of a phase 2 trial (SARC 005). Cancer *119*, 1555–1561. 10.1002/cncr.27942.

Homesley, H.D., Filiaci, V., Gibbons, S.K., Long, H.J., Cella, D., Spirtos, N.M., Morris, R.T., DeGeest, K., Lee, R., and Montag, A. (2009). A randomized phase III trial in advanced endometrial carcinoma of surgery and volume directed radiation followed by cisplatin and doxorubicin with or without paclitaxel: a Gynecologic Oncology Group study. Gynecol Oncol *112*, 543–552. 10.1016/j.ygyno.2008.11.014.

Homesley, H.D., Filiaci, V., Markman, M., Bitterman, P., Eaton, L., Kilgore, L.C., Monk, B.J., Ueland, F.R., and Gynecologic Oncology Group. (2007). Phase III trial of ifosfamide with or without paclitaxel in advanced uterine carcinosarcoma: a Gynecologic Oncology Group study. J Clin Oncol *25*, 526–531. 10.1200/JCO.2006.06.4907.

Keys, H.M., Roberts, J.A., Brunetto, V.L., Zaino, R.J., Spirtos, N.M., Bloss, J.D., Pearlman, A., Maiman, M.A., Bell, J.G., and Gynecologic Oncology Group. (2004). A phase III trial of surgery with or without adjunctive external pelvic radiation therapy in intermediate risk endometrial adenocarcinoma: a Gynecologic Oncology Group study. Gynecol Oncol *92*, 744–751. 10.1016/j.ygyno.2003.11.048.

Le, D.T., Uram, J.N., Wang, H., Bartlett, B.R., Kemberling, H., Eyring, A.D., Skora, A.D., Luber, B.S., Azad, N.S., Laheru, D., et al. (2015). PD-1 blockade in tumors with mismatch-repair deficiency. N Engl J Med *372*, 2509–2520. 10.1056/NEJMoa1500596.

Leon-Castillo, A., de Boer, S.M., Powell, M.E., Mileshkin, L.R., Mackay, H.J., Leary, A., Nijman, H.W., Singh, N., Pollock, P.M., Bessette, P., et al. (2020). Molecular classification of the PORTEC-3 trial for high-risk endometrial cancer: impact on prognosis and benefit from adjuvant therapy. J Clin Oncol *38*, 3388–3397. 10.1200/JCO.20.00549.

Lincoln, S., Blessing, J.A., Lee, R.B., and Rocereto, T.F. (2003). Activity of paclitaxel as second-line chemotherapy in endometrial carcinoma: a Gynecologic Oncology Group study. Gynecol Oncol *88*, 277–281.

Lorusso, D., Ferrandina, G., Colombo, N., Pignata, S., Pietragalla, A., Sonetto, C., Pisano, C., Lapresa, M.T., Savarese, A., Tagliaferri, P., et al. (2019). Carboplatin-paclitaxel compared to carboplatin-paclitaxel-bevacizumab in advanced or recurrent endometrial cancer: MITO END-2 — a randomized phase II trial. Gynecol Oncol *155*, 406–412. 10.1016/j.ygyno.2019.10.013.

Major, F.J., Blessing, J.A., Silverberg, S.G., Morrow, C.P., Creasman, W.T., Currie, J.L., Yordan, E., and Brady, M.F. (1993). Prognostic factors in early-stage uterine sarcoma. a Gynecologic Oncology Group study. Cancer *71*, 1702–1709.

Makker, V., Colombo, N., Herraez, A.C., Santin, A., Colomba, E., Miller, D.S., Fujiwara, K., Pignata, S., Baron, H., Ray, O.Q.A.R., et al. (2022). Lenvatinib plus pembrolizumab for advanced endometrial cancer. New Engl J Med *386*, 437–448. 10.1056/NEJMoa2108330.

Makker, V., Taylor, M.H., Aghajanian, C., Oaknin, A., Mier, J., Cohn, A.L., Romeo, M., Bratos, R., Brose, M.S., DiSimone, C., et al. (2020). Lenvatinib plus pembrolizumab in patients with advanced endometrial cancer. J Clin Oncol *38*, 2981–2992. 10.1200/JCO.19.02627.

Marabelle, A., Le, D.T., Ascierto, P.A., Di Giacomo, A.M., De Jesus-Acosta, A., Delord, J.P., Geva, R., Gottfried, M., Penel, N., Hansen, A.R., et al. (2020). Efficacy of pembrolizumab in patients with noncolorectal high microsatellite instability/mismatch repair-deficient cancer: results from the phase II KEYNOTE-158 study. J Clin Oncol *38*, 1–10. 10.1200/JCO.19.02105.

Mariani, A., Dowdy, S.C., Cliby, W.A., Gostout, B.S., Jones, M.B., Wilson, T.O., and Podratz, K.C. (2008). Prospective assessment of lymphatic dissemination in endometrial cancer: a paradigm shift in surgical staging. Gynecol Oncol *109*, 11–18. 10.1016/j.ygyno.2008.01.023.

Mariani, A., Webb, M.J., Galli, L., and Podratz, K.C. (2000a). Potential therapeutic role of para-aortic lymphadenectomy in node-positive endometrial cancer. Gynecol Oncol *76*, 348–356. 10.1006/gyno.1999.5688.

Mariani, A., Webb, M.J., Keeney, G.L., Haddock, M.G., Calori, G., and Podratz, K.C. (2000b). Low-risk corpus cancer: is lymphadenectomy or radiotherapy necessary? Am J Obstet Gynecol *182*, 1506–1519. 10.1067/mob.2000.107335.

Matei, D., Filiaci, V., Randall, M.E., Mutch, D., Steinhoff, M.M., DiSilvestro, P.A., Moxley, K.M., Kim, Y.M., Powell, M.A., O'Malley, D.M., et al. (2019). Adjuvant chemotherapy plus radiation for locally advanced endometrial cancer. N Engl J Med *380*, 2317–2326. 10.1056/NEJMoa1813181.

Miller, D.S., Filiaci, V.L., Mannel, R.S., Cohn, D.E., Matsumoto, T., Tewari, K.S., DiSilvestro, P., Pearl, M.L., Argenta, P.A., Powell, M.A., et al. (2020). Carboplatin and paclitaxel for advanced endometrial cancer: final overall survival and adverse event analysis of a phase III trial (NRG Oncology/GOG0209). J Clin Oncol *38*, 3841–3850. 10.1200/JCO.20.01076.

Nout, R.A., Smit, V.T., Putter, H., Jurgenliemk-Schulz, I.M., Jobsen, J.J., Lutgens, L.C., van der Steen-Banasik, E.M., Mens, J.W., Slot, A., Kroese, M.C., et al. (2010). Vaginal brachytherapy versus pelvic external beam radiotherapy for patients with endometrial cancer of high-intermediate risk (PORTEC-2): an open-label, non-inferiority, randomised trial. Lancet *375*, 816–823. 10.1016/S0140-6736(09)62163-2.

Nout, R.A., van de Poll-Franse, L.V., Lybeert, M.L., Warlam-Rodenhuis, C.C., Jobsen, J.J., Mens, J.W., Lutgens, L.C., Pras, B., van Putten, W.L., and Creutzberg, C.L. (2011). Long-term outcome and quality of life of patients with endometrial carcinoma treated with or without pelvic radiotherapy in the post operative radiation therapy in endometrial carcinoma 1 (PORTEC-1) trial. J Clin Oncol *29*, 1692–1700. 10.1200/JCO.2010.32.4590.

Oaknin, A., Tinker, A.V., Gilbert, L., Samouelian, V., Mathews, C., Brown, J., Barretina-Ginesta, M.P., Moreno, V., Gravina, A., Abdeddaim, C., et al. (2020). Clinical activity and safety of the anti-programmed death 1 monoclonal antibody dostarlimab for patients with recurrent or advanced mismatch repair-deficient endometrial cancer: a nonrandomized phase 1 clinical trial. JAMA Oncol *6*, 1766–1772. 10.1001/jamaoncol.2020.4515.

Omura, G.A., Blessing, J.A., Major, F., Lifshitz, S., Ehrlich, C.E., Mangan, C., Beecham, J., Park, R., and Silverberg, S. (1985). A randomized clinical trial of adjuvant adriamycin in uterine sarcomas: a Gynecologic Oncology Group study. J Clin Oncol *3*, 1240–1245. 10.1200/JCO.1985.3.9.1240.

Ott, P.A., Bang, Y.J., Berton-Rigaud, D., Elez, E., Pishvaian, M.J., Rugo, H.S., Puzanov, I., Mehnert, J.M., Aung, K.L., Lopez, J., et al. (2017). Safety and antitumor activity of pembrolizumab in advanced programmed death ligand 1-positive endometrial cancer: results from the KEYNOTE-028 study. J Clin Oncol *35*, 2535–2541. 10.1200/JCO.2017.72.5952.

Powell, M.A., Filiaci, V.L., Hensley, M.L., Huang, H.Q., Moore, K.N., Tewari, K.S., Copeland, L.J., Secord, A.A., Mutch, D.G., Santin, A., et al. (2022). Randomized phase III trial of paclitaxel and carboplatin versus paclitaxel and ifosfamide in patients with carcinosarcoma of the uterus or ovary: an NRG oncology trial. J Clin Oncol, JCO2102050. 10.1200/JCO.21.02050.

Powell, M.A., Filiaci, V.L., Rose, P.G., Mannel, R.S., Hanjani, P., Degeest, K., Miller, B.E., Susumu, N., and Ueland, F.R. (2010). Phase II evaluation of paclitaxel and carboplatin in the treatment of carcinosarcoma of the uterus: a Gynecologic Oncology Group study. J Clin Oncol *28*, 2727–2731. 10.1200/JCO.2009.26.8326.

Randall, M.E., Filiaci, V.L., McMeekin, D.S., von Gruenigen, V., Huang, H., Yashar, C.M., Mannel, R.S., Kim, J.W., Salani, R., DiSilvestro, P.A., et al. (2019). Phase III trial: adjuvant pelvic radiation therapy versus vaginal brachytherapy plus paclitaxel/carboplatin in high-intermediate and high-risk early stage endometrial cancer. J Clin Oncol *37*, 1810–1818. 10.1200/JCO.18.01575.

Randall, M.E., Filiaci, V.L., Muss, H., Spirtos, N.M., Mannel, R.S., Fowler, J., Thigpen, J.T., Benda, J.A., and Gynecologic Oncology Group, S. (2006). Randomized phase III trial of whole-abdominal irradiation versus doxorubicin and cisplatin chemotherapy in advanced endometrial carcinoma: a Gynecologic Oncology Group study. J Clin Oncol *24*, 36–44. 10.1200/JCO.2004.00.7617.

Ray-Coquard, I.L., Leary, A., Bigot, F., Montane, L., Fabbro, M., Hardy-Bessard, A.-C., Selle, F., Chakiba, C., Lortholary, A., Berton, D., et al. (2021). ROCSAN trial (GINECO-EN203b/ENGOT-EN8): a multicentric randomized phase II/III evaluating dostarlimab in combination with niraparib versus niraparib alone compared to chemotherapy in the treatment of endometrial/ovarian carcinosarcoma after at least one line of platinum based chemotherapy. J Clin Oncol *39*, TPS5604–TPS5604. 10.1200/JCO.2021.39.15_suppl.TPS5604.

Reed, N.S., Mangioni, C., Malmstrom, H., Scarfone, G., Poveda, A., Pecorelli, S., Tateo, S., Franchi, M., Jobsen, J.J., Coens, C., et al. (2008). Phase III randomised study to evaluate the role of adjuvant pelvic radiotherapy in the treatment of uterine sarcomas stages I and II: an European Organisation for Research and Treatment of Cancer

Gynaecological Cancer Group Study (protocol 55874). Eur J Cancer *44*, 808–818. 10.1016/j.ejca.2008.01.019.

Rossi, E.C., Kowalski, L.D., Scalici, J., Cantrell, L., Schuler, K., Hanna, R.K., Method, M., Ade, M., Ivanova, A., and Boggess, J.F. (2017). A comparison of sentinel lymph node biopsy to lymphadenectomy for endometrial cancer staging (FIRES trial): a multicentre, prospective, cohort study. Lancet Oncol *18*, 384–392. 10.1016/S1470-2045(17)30068-2.

Seddon, B., Strauss, S.J., Whelan, J., Leahy, M., Woll, P.J., Cowie, F., Rothermundt, C., Wood, Z., Benson, C., Ali, N., et al. (2017). Gemcitabine and docetaxel versus doxorubicin as first-line treatment in previously untreated advanced unresectable or metastatic soft-tissue sarcomas (GeDDiS): a randomised controlled phase 3 trial. Lancet Oncol *18*, 1397–1410. 10.1016/S1470-2045(17)30622-8.

Slomovitz, B.M., Filiaci, V.L., Walker, J.L., Taub, M.C., Finkelstein, K.A., Moroney, J.W., Fleury, A.C., Muller, C.Y., Holman, L.L., Copeland, L.J., et al. (2022). A randomized phase II trial of everolimus and letrozole or hormonal therapy in women with advanced, persistent or recurrent endometrial carcinoma: a GOG foundation study. Gynecol Oncol *164*, 481–491. 10.1016/j.ygyno.2021.12.031.

Slomovitz, B.M., Jiang, Y., Yates, M.S., Soliman, P.T., Johnston, T., Nowakowski, M., Levenback, C., Zhang, Q., Ring, K., Munsell, M.F., et al. (2015). Phase II study of everolimus and letrozole in patients with recurrent endometrial carcinoma. J Clin Oncol *33*, 930–936. 10.1200/JCO.2014.58.3401.

Sutton, G., Brunetto, V.L., Kilgore, L., Soper, J.T., McGehee, R., Olt, G., Lentz, S.S., Sorosky, J., and Hsiu, J.G. (2000). A phase III trial of ifosfamide with or without cisplatin in carcinosarcoma of the uterus: a Gynecologic Oncology Group study. Gynecol Oncol *79*, 147–153. 10.1006/gyno.2000.6001.

Sutton, G., Kauderer, J., Carson, L.F., Lentz, S.S., Whitney, C.W., Gallion, H., and Gynecologic Oncology Group. (2005). Adjuvant ifosfamide and cisplatin in patients with completely resected stage I or II carcinosarcomas (mixed mesodermal tumors) of the uterus: a Gynecologic Oncology Group study. Gynecol Oncol *96*, 630–634. 10.1016/j.ygyno.2004.11.022.

Thigpen, J.T., Brady, M.F., Homesley, H.D., Malfetano, J., DuBeshter, B., Burger, R.A., and Liao, S. (2004). Phase III trial of doxorubicin with or without cisplatin in advanced endometrial carcinoma: a Gynecologic Oncology Group study. J Clin Oncol *22*, 3902–3908. 10.1200/JCO.2004.02.088.

Todo, Y., Kato, H., Kaneuchi, M., Watari, H., Takeda, M., and Sakuragi, N. (2010). Survival effect of para-aortic lymphadenectomy in endometrial cancer (SEPAL study): a retrospective cohort analysis. Lancet *375*, 1165–1172. 10.1016/S0140–6736(09)62002-X.

Walker, J.L., Piedmonte, M.R., Spirtos, N.M., Eisenkop, S.M., Schlaerth, J.B., Mannel, R.S., Barakat, R., Pearl, M.L., and Sharma, S.K. (2012). Recurrence and survival after random assignment to laparoscopy versus laparotomy for comprehensive surgical staging of uterine cancer: Gynecologic Oncology Group LAP2 study. J Clin Oncol *30*, 695–700. 10.1200/JCO.2011.38.8645.

Walker, J.L., Piedmonte, M.R., Spirtos, N.M., Eisenkop, S.M., Schlaerth, J.B., Mannel, R.S., Spiegel, G., Barakat, R., Pearl, M.L., and Sharma, S.K. (2009). Laparoscopy compared with laparotomy for comprehensive surgical staging of uterine cancer: Gynecologic Oncology Group study LAP2. J Clin Oncol *27*, 5331–5336. 10.1200/JCO.2009.22.3248.

Wolfson, A.H., Brady, M.F., Rocereto, T., Mannel, R.S., Lee, Y.C., Futoran, R.J., Cohn, D.E., and Ioffe, O.B. (2007). A Gynecologic Oncology Group randomized phase III trial of whole abdominal irradiation (WAI) vs. cisplatin-ifosfamide and mesna (CIM) as post-surgical therapy in stage I-IV carcinosarcoma (CS) of the uterus. Gynecol Oncol *107*, 177–185. 10.1016/j.ygyno.2007.07.070.

Ovarian Malignancies

2

2.1 EPITHELIAL OVARIAN CANCER

2.1.1 Studies Addressing Upfront Surgery

Study: LION trial (Lymphadenectomy in Ovarian Neoplasm)

- **Citation:** (Harter et al., 2019)
- **Highlight:** No systematic lymphadenectomy during debulking surgery
- **Background:**
  - (Panici et al., 2005): Randomized controlled trial (RCT) with 427 patients showed improvement of PFS but not OS for systematic LNE vs. removal of bulky nodes in optimally debulked advanced epithelial ovarian cancer (EOC) (IIIB–IV)
  - (du Bois et al., 2010): Retrospective exploratory analysis of three AGO phase III trials suggested OS benefit of systematic LNE in advanced EOC if completely resected
- **Design:**
  - Between December 2008 and January 2012: 647 patients with advanced EOC, that is, stage IIB–IV and complete resection and pre- and intraoperatively clinically negative LNs randomized to systematic pelvic and para-aortic lymphadenectomy (LNE) vs. no LNE
  - All centers had to qualify regarding surgical skills before participation
- **Results:**
  - Median number of LNs removed: 57 (35 PLN and 22 PALN)
    - Microscopic metastases diagnosed in 56%
  - Final stage
    - Stage I–IIA: 4.6% vs. 5.2% (LNE vs. no LNE)
    - Stage IIB–IIIA: 12.7% vs. 16%
    - Stage IIIB–IV: 80.8% vs. 75.3%
  - Surgery 64 min longer with LNE
    - Higher mean blood loss (650 vs. 500 mL)
    - More transfusions (67% vs. 59%)
  - More serious complications in LNE arm
    - Re-laparotomy: 12.4% vs. 6.5% (p = 0.01)

DOI: 10.1201/9781003229711-2

- – Readmission: 8% vs. 3.1% (p = 0.006)
  - – Deaths within 60 d of surgery: 3.1% vs. 0.9% (p = 0.049)
- Postoperative carboplatin/ paclitaxel in 80% vs. 85%
- Median PFS: 25.5 months in both arms (HR 1.11 [CI = 0.92–1.34]; p = 0.29)
- Median OS: 65.5 vs. 69.2 months (HR 1.06 [CI = 0.83–1.34]; p = 0.65)
- **Conclusion:**
  - → Systematic LNE in advanced EOC does not improve PFS or OS, despite detecting and removing subclinical retroperitoneal LN; LNE should be omitted to reduce postoperative morbidity and mortality

2.1.2 Studies Addressing Adjuvant Therapy

Study: ICON1 trial (International Collaborative Ovarian Neoplasm)

- **Citation:** (Colombo et al., 2003)
- **Highlight:** Role of CT in early-stage EOC
- **Design:**
  - Between 1991 and 2000: 477 patients with early-stage ovarian cancer after surgery randomized to adjuvant CT vs. observation
  - Surgery: All visible tumor to be removed; thorough staging where possible with total hysterectomy and salpingo-oophorectomy where appropriate and omentectomy as minimum procedures
  - CT: 6 C of single-agent carboplatin or cyclophosphamide/doxorubicin/ cisplatin (CAP) or single-agent cisplatin q 3 wks recommended, but other platinum-containing regimens allowed
    - – Recommended dose of carboplatin
      - – As single agent: AUC 5
      - – In combination: AUC 4
    - – Recommended dose of cisplatin
      - – As single agent: 70 mg/m^2
      - – In CAP combination
        - – Cyclophosphamide 500 mg/m^2
        - – Doxorubicin 50 mg/m^2
        - – Cisplatin 50 mg/m^2
- **Results:**
  - Stage I: 93% (IA: 39%, IB: 11%, and IC: 40%), (73% G1 or G2); stage II: 6%; stage III: 1%
  - 5-yr OS: 79% vs. 70% (HR 0.66 [CI = 0.45–0.97]; p = 0.03) (CT vs. observation)
  - 5-yr RFS: 73% vs. 62% (HR 0.65 [CI = 0.46–0.91]; p = 0.01)
- **Conclusion:**
  - → Platinum-based CT improves survival and delays recurrence in early-stage ovarian cancer

Study: ACTION trial (Adjuvant Chemotherapy in Ovarian Neoplasm)

- **Citation:** (Trimbos et al., 2003b)
- **Highlight:** Role of CT in early-stage EOC
- **Design:**
  - 30% diagnosed in early stage; 10–50% who received surgery recur
  - Between 1990 and 2000: 448 patients with early-stage EOC randomized to platinum-based CT vs. observation
  - Surgical staging; for stage IA: USO and surgical staging permitted
    - At least careful inspection and palpation of all peritoneal surfaces, with biopsy of suspect lesions; comprehensive staging advised, including omentectomy, peritoneal washings, blind biopsy from peritoneum in pelvis (Douglas pouch, bladder, and pelvic sidewalls), paracolic gutters, and right hemidiaphragm; iliac and periaortic LN sampling (if all these requirements met → considered optimal)
  - CT: At least 4 C of platinum-based regimen; 6 C were recommended
    - Single agent and combinations allowed
    - For cisplatin, required dose: 75 mg/m^2
    - For carboplatin, required dose: 350 mg/m^2
- **Results:**
  - Stage I: 93% (IA: 35%, IB: 8%, and IC: 50%); stage II: 7%
  - Median follow-up: 5.5 yrs
  - RFS: HR 0.63 (CI = 0.43–0.92); p = 0.02
  - OS: HR 0.69 (CI = 0.44–1.08); p = 0.10
  - 1/3 of patients (n = 151) optimally staged; 2/3 not (n = 297)
    - In observation group, for optimally staged patients
      - OS improved: HR 2.31 (CI = 1.08–4.96); p = 0.03
      - RFS improved: HR 1.82 (CI = 1.02–3.24); p = 0.04
      - No such association in the CT group
    - In the CT group, for non-optimally staged patients
      - OS improved: HR 1.75 (CI = 1.04–2.95); p = 0.03
      - RFS improved: HR 1.78 (CI = 1.15–2.77); p = 0.009
      - In optimally staged patients, no benefit of CT
- **Conclusion:**
  - → Adjuvant CT associated with improved RFS in early-stage ovarian cancer; benefit seemed to be limited to patients with non-optimal staging (i.e., patients with higher risk of unappreciated disease)

Study: ICON/ACTION merger

- **Citation:** (Trimbos et al., 2003a)
- **Highlight:** Role of CT in early-stage EOC
- **Design:**
  - Initially planned for ICON1 to enroll 2,000 patients
  - During accrual period, survival in no-adjuvant CT better than anticipated and slow accrual → in June 1999, decision to combine ICON1 and ACTION

- Preplanned combined analysis of two parallel RCTs (ICON1 and EORTEC–ACTION)
- 925 patients (477 in ICON1; 448 in ACTION) with early-stage ovarian cancer after surgery randomized to platinum-based adjuvant CT vs. observation
- **Results:**
  - Median follow-up: 4 yrs
  - 5-yr OS: 82% vs. 74% (HR 0.67 [CI = 0.5–0.9]; p = 0.008) (CT vs. observation)
  - 5-yr RFS: 76% vs. 65% (HR 0.64 [CI = 0.5–0.82]; p = 0.001)
  - No difference in size of effect of CT in any subgroup
    - Pretreatment age, tumor stage, histologic cell type, and grade
- **Conclusion:**
  - → Platinum-based adjuvant CT improved overall and RFS in early-stage ovarian cancer

Study: GOG 157

- **Citation:** (Bell et al., 2006)
- **Highlight:** 3 vs. 6 C in high-risk early-stage EOC
- **Design:**
  - 427 patients with stage IA G3 (or clear cell), IB G3 (or clear cell), stage IC, and completely resected stage II EOC randomized to 3 vs. 6 C of carboplatin and paclitaxel
  - Paclitaxel: 175 mg/m^2 over 3 hrs; carboplatin: AUC 7.5 over 30 min q 3 wks
- **Results:**
  - Median follow-up: 6.8 yrs
  - Grade 3 or 4 neurotoxicity: 4/211 (2%) vs. 24/212 (11%); p < 0.01 (3 vs. 6 C)
  - Significantly more anemia and granulocytopenia with 6 C
  - Recurrence rate for 6 C 24% lower (HR 0.761 [CI = 0.51–1.13]; p = 0.18); estimated recurrence rate in 5 yrs: 25.4% vs. 20.1%
  - Death rate: HR 1.02 (CI = 0.662–1.57)
- **Conclusion:**
  - → 6 C of carboplatin/ paclitaxel do not alter recurrence rate in high-risk early-stage EOC but have more toxicity compared to 3 C

Study: ICON2

- **Citation:** (ICON2 (1998): randomized trial of single-agent carboplatin against three-drug combination of CAP (cyclophosphamide, doxorubicin, and cisplatin) in women with ovarian cancer (ICON Collaborators. International Collaborative Ovarian Neoplasm Study, 1998)
- **Highlight:** Single-agent carboplatin vs. CAP in advanced EOC
- **Design:**
  - 1,526 patients with advanced ovarian cancer randomized to cyclophosphamide 500 mg/m^2, doxorubicin 50 mg/m^2, and cisplatin

50 mg/m² (CAP) q 3 wks × 6 C vs. single-agent carboplatin AUC 5 q 3 wks × 6 C

- **Results:**
  - No difference in OS
    - Median survival: 33 months
    - 2-yr survival: 60% for both groups
    - No difference in effectiveness in different subgroups of age, stage, residual disease, grade, histology, and center
  - CAP more toxic
    - More alopecia, leukopenia, and nausea with CAP
    - More thrombocytopenia with carboplatin
- **Conclusion:**
  - → Single-agent carboplatin with dose calculated by AUC is safe, effective, and an appropriate standard of treatment for advanced ovarian cancer

Study: GOG 111

- **Citation:** (McGuire et al., 1996)
- **Highlight:** Cisplatin plus paclitaxel or cyclophosphamide for advanced EOC
- **Design:**
  - 386 patients with advanced stage ovarian cancer and residual disease > 1 cm (suboptimally debulked) randomized to cisplatin 75 mg/m² plus cyclophosphamide 750 mg/m² q 3wks × 6 C vs. cisplatin 75 mg/m² plus paclitaxel 135 mg/m² over 24 hrs q 3 wks × 6 C
- **Results:**
  - Toxicities
    - Alopecia grade 2: 54% vs. 27% (taxane vs. cyclophosphamide)
    - Neutropenia ≥ grade 3: 92% vs. 83%
      - However, incidence of febrile neutropenia low, consistent with brevity of paclitaxel-induced myelosuppression
    - Fever ≥ grade 3: 0% vs. 3–4%
    - Allergic reactions ≥ grade 3: 0% vs. 4%
  - 87% vs. 78% completed 6 C
  - 73% vs. 60% of 216 women with measurable disease responded (p = 0.01)
  - Frequency of surgically verified CR similar
  - Median PFS: 18 vs. 13 months (p < 0.001)
  - Median OS: 38 vs. 24 months (p < 0.001)
- **Conclusion:**
  - → Incorporating paclitaxel into first-line CT improves PFS and OS in incompletely resected stage III and IV ovarian cancer

Study: Intergroup trial

- **Citation:** (Piccart et al., 2000)
- **Highlight:** Cisplatin plus paclitaxel or cyclophosphamide for advanced EOC

- **Design:**
  - Based on GOG 111, European and Canadian investigators launched confirmatory trial with broader eligibility criteria
  - 680 patients with advanced ovarian cancer randomized to cisplatin plus cyclophosphamide vs. cisplatin plus paclitaxel over 3 hrs (instead of 24 hrs as in GOG 111)
    - Stage IIB, IIC, III, and IV; within 8 wks of optimal or suboptimal cytoreduction
- **Results:**
  - Median follow-up: 38.5 months
  - ORR: 59% vs. 45% (p = 0.01)
    - CR: 41% vs. 27% (p = 0.01)
  - Median PFS: 15.5 vs. 11.5 months (p = 0.0005); 26% reduction in progression rate (HR 0.74; CI = 0.63–0.88) qualitatively unchanged when stage, histologic type, and residual disease considered
  - Median OS: 35.6 vs. 25.8 months (p = 0.0016); 27% reduction in death rate (HR 0.73; CI = 0.6–0.89) qualitatively unchanged when stage, histologic type, and residual disease considered
- **Conclusion:**
  - → Strong and confirmatory evidence to support paclitaxel–cisplatin as new standard of treatment for advanced ovarian cancer

Study: GOG 158

- **Citation:** (Ozols et al., 2003)
- **Highlight:** Non-inferiority trial of carbo/taxane vs. cis/taxane
- **Design:**
  - In non-randomized trials, carboplatin and paclitaxel less toxic than cisplatin and paclitaxel and highly active; here, non-inferiority trial
  - 792 patients with advanced ovarian cancer optimally resected (≤1 cm) randomized to cisplatin 75 mg/m^2 plus paclitaxel 135 mg/m^2 over 24 hrs vs. carboplatin AUC 7.5 plus paclitaxel 175 mg/m^2 over 3 hrs
- **Results:**
  - Toxicities
    - GI grade ≥ 3: 23% vs. 10% (cis vs. carbo)
    - GU grade ≥ 3: 3% vs. 1%
    - Metabolic grade ≥ 3: 8% vs. 3%
    - Leukopenia grade 4: 12% vs. 6%
    - Thrombocytopenia grade ≥ 3: 5% vs. 39%
    - Neurologic toxicities similar (grade 3: 8% vs 7%)
  - Median PFS: 19.4 vs. 20.7 months; RR of progression for carbo 0.88 (CI = 0.75–1.03)
  - Median OS: 48.7 vs. 57.4 months; RR for death 0.85 (CI = 0.7–1.02)
- **Conclusion:**
  - → Carboplatin plus taxane results in less toxicity, easier to administer, and not inferior when compared with cisplatin plus taxane in advanced ovarian cancer

Study: ICON3

- **Citation:** (International Collaborative Ovarian Neoplasm, 2002)
- **Highlight:** Carbo/Taxol vs. CAP or single-agent carbo
- **Design:**
  - February 1995 to October 1998: 2,074 patients with ovarian cancer randomized to paclitaxel 175 mg/m^2 over 3 hrs plus carboplatin AUC 6 vs. control; control (cyclophosphamide 500 mg/m^2, doxorubicin 50 mg/m^2, cisplatin 50 mg/m^2 [CAP] or single-agent carboplatin AUC 6) chosen by patient and clinician before randomization
- **Results:**
  - Toxicities
    - Paclitaxel plus carboplatin associated with more alopecia, fever, sensory neuropathy than carboplatin alone, and more sensory neuropathy than CAP
    - CAP associated with more fever than paclitaxel plus carboplatin
  - Median follow-up: 51 months
  - Median PFS: 17.3 vs. 16.1 months (paclitaxel plus carboplatin vs. control)
  - Median OS: 36.1 vs. 35.4 months
- **Conclusion:**
  - → Single-agent carboplatin and CAP as effective as paclitaxel plus carboplatin as first-line CT for ovarian cancer; favorable toxicity profile of carboplatin

Study: GOG 182/ICON5

- **Citation:** (Bookman et al., 2009)
- **Highlight:** Addition of third cytotoxic agent to adjuvant therapy
- **Design:**
  - To determine if addition of another cytotoxic agent to carboplatin/ paclitaxel improves OS and PFS
  - 4,312 patients with stage III and IV ovarian cancer optimally or suboptimally cytoreduced randomized to five arms
    - Arm 1 (reference): Carboplatin AUC 6 and paclitaxel 175 mg/m^2 over 3 hrs on day 1 q 3 wks × 8 C
    - Arm 2: Carboplatin AUC 5 and paclitaxel 175 mg/m^2 over 3 hrs on day 1 plus gemcitabine 800 mg/m^2 over 30 min on days 1 and 8 q 3 wks × 8 C
    - Arm 3: Carboplatin AUC 5 and paclitaxel 175 mg/m^2 over 3 hrs on day 1 q 3 wks × 8 C plus pegylated liposomal doxorubicin (PLD) 30 mg/m^2 on day 1 for C 1, 3, 5, and 7
    - Arm 4: Carboplatin AUC 5 on day 3 and topotecan 1.25 mg/m^2 on days 1, 2, and 3 q 3 wks × 4 C, followed by carboplatin AUC 6 on day 1 and paclitaxel 175 mg/m^2 over 3 hrs on day 1 × 4 C
    - Arm 5: Carboplatin AUC 6 on day 8 and gemcitabine 1,000 mg/m^2 over on days 1 and 8 q 3 wks × 4 C, followed by carboplatin AUC 6 on day 1 and paclitaxel 175 mg/m^2 over 3 hrs on day 1 × 4 C

- Stratified by center, diameter of residual tumor, and intent to perform interval cytoreduction (about 7–8% in each arm)
- **Results:**
  - 79% completed 8 C
  - No improvements in PFS (HR from 0.984 to 1.066) or OS (HR 0.952 to 1.114)
    - Also, in subgroup analysis defined by size of residual disease—no benefit in any subgroup
- **Conclusion:**
  - → Addition of third cytotoxic agent did not provide any benefit over standard carboplatin/ paclitaxel in PFS or OS in optimally and suboptimally cytoreduced patients

Study: GOG 132

- **Citation:** (Muggia et al., 2000)
- **Highlight:** Single-agent cisplatin vs. single-agent Taxol vs. cisplatin/Taxol in suboptimally debulked EOC
- **Design:**
  - 648 patients with suboptimally debulked EOC randomized to cisplatin 100 mg/m^2 q 3 wks × 6 C vs. paclitaxel 200 mg/m^2 over 24 hrs q 3 wks × 6 C vs. paclitaxel 135 mg/m^2 plus cisplatin 75 mg/m^2 q 3 wks × 6 C
- **Results:**
  - Monotherapies discontinued more frequently
    - Cisplatin because of toxicity or refusal: 17%
    - Paclitaxel because of progression: 20%
  - Toxicities
    - Neutropenia, fever, and alopecia more severe with paclitaxel-containing regimens
    - Anemia, thrombocytopenia, neurotoxicity, nephrotoxicity, and GI toxicity more severe with cisplatin-containing regimens
  - ORR: 42% vs. 67% ($p < 0.001$) (single-agent paclitaxel vs. cisplatin regimens)
  - Relative hazard (RH) of progression or death greater for paclitaxel compared to cisplatin regimens: RH = 1.41 (CI = 1.15–1.73); $p < 0.001$
    - But did not differ significantly between the two cisplatin regimens
  - Relative to cisplatin, death rate for paclitaxel higher (RH = 1.15 [CI = 0.929–1.42]) and for combination slightly lower (RH = 0.99 [CI = 0.795–1.23]; not statistically significant)
- **Conclusion:**
  - → Cisplatin alone or in combination with superior response rates and PFS compared to paclitaxel; OS similar in all arms; combination with better toxicity profile; therefore, combination of cisplatin and paclitaxel remains preferred initial treatment

Study: MITO-2

- **Citation:** (Pignata et al., 2011)
- **Highlight:** Carbo/doxil vs. carbo/Taxol
- **Design:**
  - 820 patients with stage IC to IV, age ≤75, ECOG score ≤2 randomized to carboplatin AUC 5 plus paclitaxel 175 mg/m^2 vs. carboplatin AUC 5 plus PLD 30 mg/m^2 q 3 wks × 6 C
  - 632 events in 820 enrolled patients would have 80% power to detect 0.8 HR of PFS
    - Occurrence of PFS events slowed down; decision for analysis with 556 events
- **Results:**
  - Median follow-up: 40 months
  - Less neurotoxicity and alopecia, but more hematologic AE with carbo/PLD
  - No difference in QoL after 3 and 6 C
  - Median PFS: 19 vs. 16.8 months (carbo/PLD vs. carbo/Taxol) (HR = 0.95 [CI = 0.81–1.13]; p = 0.58)
  - Median OS: 61.6 vs. 53.2 months (HR = 0.89 [CI = 0.72–1.12]; p = 0.32)
- **Conclusion:**
  - → Carbo/PLD not superior to carbo/Taxol, which remains first-line CT for advanced ovarian cancer; however, given observed CIs and different toxicities, carbo/PLD could be considered alternative to standard treatment

Study: JGOG 3016

- **Citation:** (Katsumata et al., 2009)
- **Highlight:** Dose-dense Taxol
- **Design:**
  - 631 patients with stage II, III, and IV EOC after optimal or suboptimal cytoreduction randomized to paclitaxel 180 mg/m^2 over 3 hrs plus carboplatin AUC 6 on day 1 q 3 wks × 6 C vs. dose-dense paclitaxel 80 mg/m^2 over 1 hr on days 1, 8, and 15 plus carboplatin AUC 6 on day 1 q 3 wks
    - Interval debulking surgery (IDS) after 2–4 C; secondary debulking or second-look surgery after 6 C or both allowed
    - Responding patents received three additional cycles
- **Results:**
  - Stage II 18%, stage III 66%, and stage IV 15.5%
  - Primary debulking 89%, IDS 10%, secondary/second look 15%
  - Optimally resected 46%; suboptimally debulked 54%
  - 165/321 (51% of dose dense) and 117/319 (37% of conventional) discontinued treatment early

- – For toxicity in 113 vs. 69 patients (dose dense vs. conventional)
- Toxicities
  - – Neutropenia: 92% vs. 88%
  - – Grade 3 and 4 anemia: 69% vs. 44% (p < 0.0001)
- Median PFS: 28.0 vs. 17.2 months (p = 0.0015)
- 3-yr OS: 72.1% vs. 65.1% (p = 0.03)
- **Conclusion:**
  - → Dose-dense paclitaxel plus carboplatin improved survival compared to conventional treatment and is new treatment option in advanced EOC

Study: JGOG 3016

- **Citation:** (Katsumata et al., 2013)
- **Highlight:** Long-term follow-up
- **Results:**
  - Median follow-up: 76.8 months
  - Median PFS: 28.2 vs 17.5 months (p = 0.0037)
  - Median OS: 100.5 vs 62.2 months (p = 0.039)

Study: MITO-7

- **Citation:** (Pignata et al., 2014)
- **Highlight:** Weekly carbo/Taxol vs. 3-weekly carbo/Taxol
- **Design:**
  - To confirm JGOG findings on dose-dense Taxol
  - 810 patients with stage IC–IV, chemo-naïve randomized to carboplatin AUC 6 plus paclitaxel 175 mg/m^2 q 3 wks × 6 C vs. carboplatin AUC 2 plus paclitaxel 60 mg/m^2 q wk × 18 wks
- **Results:**
  - Median follow-up: 17.3–18.3 months
  - FACT-O/TOI scores worsened with every cycle in 3-weekly regimen, while for weekly regimen scores remained stable after transient worsening at week 1 (p < 0.0001)
  - Grade 3–4 neutropenia: 50% vs. 42% (3-weekly vs. weekly)
  - Febrile neutropenia: 3% vs. 0.5%
  - Grade 3–4 thrombocytopenia: 7% vs. 1%
  - ≥ Grade 2 neuropathy: 17% vs. 6%
  - Median PFS: 17.3 vs. 18.3 months (p = 0.66)
- **Conclusion:**
  - → Weekly regimen of carbo/Taxol might be reasonable option for first line in advanced ovarian cancer

Study: GOG 262

- **Citation:** (Chan et al., 2016)
- **Highlight:** Carbo/Taxol (+ possibly BEV) vs. carbo/dose-dense Taxol (+ possibly BEV)

- **Design:**
  - 692 patients with newly diagnosed, incompletely resected stage III or any stage IV EOC ovarian cancer prospectively stratified according to whether or not they opted to receive BEV and randomized to paclitaxel 175 mg/m^2 q 3 wks plus carboplatin AUC 6 × 6 C vs. paclitaxel 80 mg/m^2 q wk plus carboplatin AUC 6 × 6 C
    - After closure of GOG 252, patients with stage II or III with optimally resected EOC (≤1 cm) also included
    - Also, patients who underwent NACT
- **Results:**
  - Stage II: 3%, stage III: 67%, and stage IV: 30%
  - 84% of patients opted to receive BEV
  - 13% opted for NACT
  - Toxicities
    - With dose-dense paclitaxel
      - Higher rate of grade 3 or 4 anemia (36% vs. 16%)
      - Higher rate of grade 2–4 sensory neuropathy (26% vs. 18%)
      - Lower rate of grade 3 or 4 neutropenia (72% vs. 83%)
  - Median PFS: 14.7 vs. 14.0 months (dose-dense vs. q 3 wks) (p = 0.18)
    - For patients who did not receive BEV, median PFS: 14.2 vs. 10.3 months (p = 0.03)
    - For patients who received BEV, median PFS: 14.9 vs. 14.7 months (p = 0.6)
  - Median OS: 40.2 vs. 39 months
- **Conclusion:**
  - → Overall, weekly paclitaxel compared to q 3 wks did not prolong PFS among ovarian cancer patients

Study: ICON8

- **Citation:** (Clamp et al., 2019)
- **Highlight:** Dose-dense paclitaxel
- **Background:** JGOG3016 showed PFS and OS benefit of dose-dense weekly paclitaxel in Japanese population; here, randomized trial in mainly European population
- **Design:**
  - 1,566 patients with stage IC grade 3 to stage IV EOC randomized to arm 1: Carboplatin AUC 5/6 and paclitaxel 175 mg/m^2 q 3 wks; arm 2: Carboplatin AUC 5/6 and paclitaxel 80 mg/m^2 q 1 wk; arm 3: Carboplatin AUC 2 and paclitaxel 80 mg/m^2 q 1 wk
  - Patients entered after primary surgery or received NACT
  - Primary intention-to-treat analysis compared arm 2 vs. arm 1 and arm 3 vs. arm 1
- **Results:**
  - 72% serous histology
  - 92% ECOG performance status 0/1

- 48% upfront surgery; 50% IDS; 3% inoperable
- 72%, 60%, and 63% completed six cycles in arms 1, 2, and 3
- 90%, 89%, and 85% completed six cycles of carboplatin in arms 1, 2, and 3
- AEs
  - Grade 3/4 toxicity (mainly uncomplicated neutropenia): 42%, 62%, and 53%
  - Febrile neutropenia: 4%, 6%, and 3%
  - ≥Grade 2 neuropathy: 27%, 24%, and 22%
- No significant increase in PFS
  - Arm 2 vs. 1 (p = 0.35)
  - Arm 3 vs. 1 (p = 0.51)
  - Median PFS: 17.7, 20.8, and 21.0 months
- **Conclusion:**
  - → Weekly paclitaxel can be delivered successfully as first-line treatment for ovarian cancer, but does not significantly improve PFS

2.1.3 Studies Addressing Intraperitoneal Chemotherapy

Study: GOG 104

- **Citation:** (Alberts et al., 1996)
- **Highlight:** Cyclophosphamide plus ip cisplatin vs. iv cisplatin in stage III EOC
- **Design:**
  - 546 patients with stage III EOC within 4–6 wks after resection of all tumor >2 cm randomized to 6 C iv cyclophosphamide (600 mg/m^2) plus ip cisplatin (100 mg/m^2) vs. 6 C iv cyclophosphamide plus iv cisplatin (100 mg/m^2) q 3 wks
- **Results:**
  - Toxicities
    - Moderate-to-severe tinnitus: 7% vs. 14% (p < 0.001) (ip vs. iv)
    - Hearing loss: 5% vs. 15%
    - Neuromuscular toxic effects: 15% vs. 25%
    - Granulocytopenia: 56% vs. 69% (p = 0.002)
    - Leukopenia: 40% vs. 50% (p = 0.04)
  - Median survival: 49 vs. 41 months
  - Mortality lower in ip group: HR = 0.76 (CI = 0.61–0.96); p = 0.02
- **Conclusion:**
  - → IP cisplatin improves survival and has fewer toxic effects in stage III EOC with residual tumor <2 cm

Study: GOG 114

- **Citation:** (Markman et al., 2001)
- **Highlight:** Taxane plus iv vs. iv/ip platinum in stage III EOC

- 462 patients with stage III EOC and small-volume residual disease (≤ 1 cm optimally resected) randomized to paclitaxel (135 mg/m^2 over 24 hrs) plus iv cisplatin (75 mg/m^2) q 3 wks × 6 C vs. iv carboplatin (AUC 9) q 4 wks × 2 C, then iv paclitaxel 135 mg/m^2 over 24 hrs followed by ip cisplatin (100 mg/m^2) q 3 wks × 6 C
- 86% vs. 71% patients completed 6 C (iv vs. iv/ip)
- Toxicities
  - Grade 4 neutropenia: 13% vs. 28%
  - Grade 4 thrombocytopenia: 1% vs. 24%
  - Grade 4 GI toxicities: 8% vs. 20%
  - Metabolic toxicities: 1% vs. 3%
  - → 18% received ≤ 2 C of ip therapy
- Median PFS: 22 vs. 28 months (p = 0.01)
- Median OS: 52 vs. 63 months (p = 0.05)
- **Conclusion:**
  - → Moderately high iv carboplatin followed by iv paclitaxel and ip cisplatin with significant improvement in PFS
  - Because of borderline improvement in OS and greater toxicity, not recommended for routine use; however, need for further investigation in small-volume residual EOC

Study: GOG 172

- **Citation:** (Armstrong et al., 2006)
- **Highlight:** IV vs. iv/ip in stage III EOC
- **Design:**
  - 415 patients with stage III EOC optimally resected (≤ 1 cm) randomized to iv paclitaxel (135 mg/m^2 over 24 hrs) followed by iv cisplatin (75 mg/m^2 on day 2) q 3 wks × 6 C vs. iv paclitaxel (135 mg/m^2 over 24 hrs) followed by ip cisplatin (100 mg/m^2 on day 2) and ip paclitaxel (60 mg/m^2 on day 8) q 3 wks × 6 C
- **Results:**
  - Toxicities more common in ip group
    - Grade 3 and 4 pain: 11% vs. 1% (p < 0.001) (ip vs. iv)
    - Fatigue: 18% vs. 4% (p < 0.001)
    - Hematologic
      - Leukopenia: 76% vs. 64% (p < 0.001)
      - Thrombocytopenia: 12% vs. 4% (p0.002)
    - GI: 46% vs. 24% (p < 0.001)
    - Metabolic: 27% vs. 7% (p < 0.001)
    - Neurologic: 19% vs. 9% (p = 0.001)
  - 42% in ip group completed 6 C
  - QoL significantly worse in ip group before C 4 (p < 0.001) and 3–6 wks after treatment (p = 0.009), but not 1 yr after treatment (p = 0.56)
  - Median PFS: 23.8 vs. 18.3 months (p = 0.05)

- For gross residual disease (≤1 cm): 18.3 vs. 15.4 months, RR: 0.81 (CI = 0.62–1.05)
- For no visible residual disease: 37.6 vs. 35.2 months, RR: 0.8 (CI = 0.54–1.21)
- Median OS: 65.6 vs. 49.7 months (p = 0.03)
- **Conclusion:**
  - → IV paclitaxel plus ip cisplatin and paclitaxel improves survival in optimally debulked stage III EOC

Study: GOG 252

- **Citation:** (Walker et al., 2019)
- **Highlight:** IV carbo vs. ip carbo vs. ip cis, all plus BEV therapy and maintenance
- **Design:**
  - 1,560 patients with stage II and stage III EOC optimally resected randomized to arm 1: iv paclitaxel 80 mg/m² over 1 hr on days 1, 8, and 15 and iv carboplatin AUC 6 over 30 min on day 1 q 3 wks × 6 C, then followed by BEV beginning on C 2 × 22 C vs. arm 2: iv paclitaxel 80 mg/m² over 1 hr on days 1, 8, and 15 and ip carboplatin AUC 6 on day 1 q 3 wks × 6 C, then followed by BEV beginning on C 2 × 22 C vs. arm 3: iv paclitaxel 135 mg/m² over 3 hrs on day 1, and ip cisplatin 75 mg/m² on day 2, and ip paclitaxel 60 mg/m² on day 8 q 3 wks × 6 C, then followed by BEV beginning on C 2 × 22 C
  - Arm 1: iv carbo (reference arm); arm 2: ip carbo; arm 3: ip cisplatin
  - Dosing differences compared to GOG 172
    - Cisplatin dose reduced (100 → 75)
    - Infusion time reduced (24 hrs → 3 hrs)
    - All outpatient infusions
    - Addition of BEV
    - Comparison of dose-dense paclitaxel with carbo iv AUC 6 (GOG 262/JGOG)
    - Additional arm with ip carbo and dose-dense paclitaxel
- **Results:**
  - Stage II: 10%; stage III: 84%
  - At least 6 C of platinum-containing CT
    - In arms 1 and 2: 90%
    - In arm 3: 84%
  - At least 6 C taxane
    - Arms 1 and 3: 87%; arm 2: 88%
  - Crossover to iv only, in 16% of ip carbo patients and 28% of ip cisplatin
  - Toxicities
    - Neutropenia ≥ grade 3: 72% in iv carbo, 68% in ip carbo, and 64% in ip cisplatin
    - Thrombocytopenia ≥ grade 3: 18% in iv carbo, 15% in ip carbo, and 11% in ip cisplatin

- – HTN ≥ grade 3: 12% in iv carbo, 14% in ip carbo, and 20.5% in ip cisplatin
- – N/V ≥ grade 3: 5% in iv carbo, 5% in ip carbo, and 11% in ip cisplatin
- – Fistula ≥ grade 3: 5% in iv carbo, 4% in ip carbo, and 4% in ip cisplatin
- – Sensory neuropathy ≥ grade 3: 5.7% in iv carbo, 4.5% in ip carbo, and 5.5% in ip cisplatin; up to 30% grade 2
- Median PFS
  - – For ≤1 cm
    - – 26.9 vs. 28.7 vs. 27.8 months (iv carbo [reference] vs. ip carbo vs. ip cisplatin) (p = 0.416 and 0.727)
  - – No visible disease
    - – 35.9 vs. 38.8 vs. 35.5 months
  - – CT imaging was required q 6 months for surveillance (not required in GOG 114 and 172)
- Survival data not available yet
- **Conclusion**:
  - → All arms with 'excessive toxicity'; neurotoxicity similar in all arms, IP cisplatin increases BEV-associated HTN; no changes in current treatment recommendations until survival data available
    - – Dose reductions of paclitaxel and cisplatin and crossover may have compromised efficacy
    - – Dose-dense paclitaxel may improve efficacy and may allow to abandon ip CT
    - – BEV interactions may have clouded analysis

Study: Dutch HIPEC trial

- **Citation:** (van Driel et al., 2018)
- **Highlight:** Hyperthermic intraperitoneal chemotherapy (HIPEC) after neoadjuvant CT and IDS
- **Design:**
  - 245 patients with stage III EOC and at least SD after three C of neoadjuvant CT with carboplatin AUC 5 or 6 and paclitaxel 175 mg/m^2 randomized to HIPEC (cisplatin 100 mg/m^2 for 90 min) vs. no HIPEC
  - Randomization at time of surgery, if complete or optimal debulking seemed possible
  - Three additional C of adjuvant CT with carboplatin/ paclitaxel administered
- **Results:**
  - HR of disease recurrence or death: 0.66 (CI = 0.50–0.87); p = 0.003
  - Median recurrence-free interval: 10.7 vs. 14.2 months (surgery vs. surgery + HIPEC)
  - At median follow-up of 4.7 yrs: 62% vs. 50% had died (HR: 0.67 [CI = 0.48–0.94]; p = 0.02)
  - Median OS: 33.9 vs. 45.7 months
  - ≥ Grade 3 AEs: 25% vs. 27% (p = 0.76)

- **Conclusion**:
  - → Addition of HIPEC to IDS after NACT for stage III EOC resulted in longer RFS and OS and similar rate of side effects

Study: Sloan HIPEC trial for recurrent EOC

- **Citation:** (Zivanovic et al., 2021)
- **Highlight:** HIPEC at the time of secondary debulking surgery
- **Design:**
  - In a randomized phase II trial, 98 patients underwent secondary cytoreduction with or without carboplatin HIPEC (800 mg/m^2 for 90 min) followed by five to six C of iv platinum-based CT
- **Results:**
  - Complete gross resection in 82% vs. 94% (HIPEC vs. standard)
  - Bowel resections in 37% vs. 65%
  - No difference in length of stay or postoperative toxicity
  - Median PFS: 12.3 vs. 15.7 months (p = 0.05)
  - Median OS: 52.5 vs. 59.7 months
- **Conclusion:**
  - → HIPEC with carboplatin well tolerated but did not result in superior outcomes

2.1.4 Studies Addressing First-Line Maintenance Treatment

Study: GOG 178

- **Citation:** (Markman et al., 2003)
- **Highlight:** 3 vs. 12 C single-agent Taxol maintenance
- **Design:**
  - 262 patients with stage III and IV ovarian cancer who have been treated with 5–6 C of a platinum/paclitaxel regimen and attained CR randomized to 3 C single-agent paclitaxel 175 mg/m^2 over 3 hrs q 4 wks vs. 12 C single-agent paclitaxel 175 mg/m^2 over 3 hrs q 4 wks
- **Results:**
  - Toxicities
    - Peripheral neuropathy grade 2: 14% vs. 18%; grade 3: 1% vs. 5% (3 vs. 12 C)
  - Median PFS: 21 vs. 28 months (HR 2.31 [CI = 1.08–4.94]; p = 0.0023)
  - Because of protocol-specified early termination boundary of p = 0.005, trial was discontinued
  - No difference in OS
- **Conclusion:**
  - → 12 C of single-agent paclitaxel in women with advanced ovarian cancer who attain CR in response to initial platinum/paclitaxel CT significantly prolong PFS

Study: GOG 218

- **Citation:** (Burger et al., 2011)
- **Highlight:** Carbo/Taxol ± BEV initiation or throughout therapy
- **Design:**
  - 1,873 patients with newly diagnosed stage III (incompletely resectable) or any stage IV EOC randomized to paclitaxel 175 mg/m^2 plus carboplatin AUC 6 q 3 wks × 6 C (control) vs. paclitaxel 175 mg/m^2 plus carboplatin AUC 6 q 3 wks × 6 C plus BEV (15 mg/kg) in C 2–6 (BEV initiation treatment) vs. paclitaxel 175 mg/m^2 plus carboplatin AUC 6 q 3 wks × 6 C plus BEV (15 mg/kg) in C 2–22 (BEV throughout treatment)
    - Because of competing trials, optimally debulked stage III disease initially excluded but after protocol modification permitted
- **Results:**
  - Stage III, optimally cytoreduced: 34%, stage III, suboptimally cytoreduced: 40%; stage IV: 25.7%
  - Toxicities
    - Hypertension requiring medication: 7.2% vs. 16.5% vs. 22.9%
    - GI perforation requiring intervention: 1.2% vs. 2.8% vs. 2.6%
  - Median PFS: 10.3 vs. 11.2 vs. 14.1 months (control vs. initiation vs. throughout)
  - HR for progression or death relative to control 0.908 (CI = 0.795–1.040) and 0.717 (CI = 0.625–0.824; p < 0.001) for initiation and throughout
  - No significant difference in OS
- **Conclusion:**
  - → Use of BEV during and up to 10 months after carboplatin and paclitaxel prolongs PFS by about 4 months in advanced EOC

Study: ICON7

- **Citation:** (Perren et al., 2011)
- **Highlight:** Carbo/Taxol ± BEV throughout therapy
- **Design:**
  - 1,528 patients with ovarian cancer, high-risk early stage (stage I or IIA clear cell or G 3) or advanced stage (stages IIB–IV) randomized to carboplatin AUC 5 or 6 and paclitaxel 175 mg/m^2 q 3 wks × 6 C vs. carboplatin AUC 5 or 6 and paclitaxel 175 mg/m^2 q 3 wks × 6 C plus BEV (7.5 mg/kg) given concurrently for 5 or 6 C and continued for additional 12 cycles
- **Results:**
  - Stage I/IIA: 10%; stage IIB/IIC: 9%; stage III: 67%; stage IV: 13%
  - Inoperable: 1%; suboptimally debulked: 25%; optimally debulked: 73%
  - Toxicities
    - HTN grade ≥2: 2% vs. 18%
    - Thromboembolic events: 3% vs. 7%
    - GI perforations: 1/753 vs. 10/745
  - 91% and 94% received six cycles (standard vs. BEV); 62% received 18 cycles

- PFS (restricted mean) at 36 months: 20.3 vs. 21.8 months (standard vs. BEV); HR for progression or death with BEV: 0.81 (C = 0.7–0.94; p = 0.004)
  - Nonproportional hazards detected (i.e., treatment effect not consistent over time), with maximum effect at 12 months (end of planned BEV treatment) and diminishing by 24 months
- PFS (restricted mean) at 42 months: 22.4 vs. 24.1 months (p = 0.04)
- In patients at high risk of progression, benefit greater: PFS (restricted mean) at 42 months 14.5 vs. 18.1 months, with median OS: 28.8 vs. 36.6 months
  - Definition of high risk for progression
    - Stage IV
    - Suboptimally debulked stage III
- **Conclusion:**
  - → BEV improved PFS
  - Benefits in PFS and OS greater among those at high risk for progression

Study: ICON7

- **Citation:** (Oza et al., 2015)
  - **Highlight:** Long-term follow-up
  - **Design:**
  - Definition of high risk for progression
    - Stage IV
    - Suboptimally debulked stage III
    - Inoperable stage III
  - Results with nonproportional hazards; therefore, difference in restricted mean survival time used
- **Results:**
  - No OS benefit; restricted mean OS: 44.6 vs. 45.5 months
    - In poor-prognosis disease
      - Restricted mean survival time: 34.5 vs. 39.3 months (p = 0.03)
  - No difference in PFS
- **Conclusion:**
  - → BEV added to platinum-based CT did not increase OS in the studied group as a whole
  - However, in subgroup of poor-prognosis patients, survival benefit recorded (concordant with PFS results from ICON7 and GOG 218)

Study: BOOST

- **Citation:** (Pfisterer et al., 2021)
- **Highlight:** BEV treatment duration
- **Design:**
  - 927 patients with stage IIB–IV ovarian cancer s/p primary cytoreductive surgery followed by six C carboplatin AUC 5, paclitaxel 175 mg/m^2 and BEV 15 mg/kg randomized to 15 vs. 30 months BEV maintenance

- **Results:**
  - Median PFS: 24.2 vs. 26 months (HR 0.99; p = 0.9) (15 vs. 30 months)
  - Restricted mean PFS: 39.5 vs. 39.3 months
  - Median OS: 54.3 vs. 60 months (HR 1.04; p = 0.68)
  - Restricted mean OS: 60.4 vs. 60.8 months
  - Serious AEs: 11% vs 14%; hypertension (2.7% vs. 4.5%), thromboembolic event (2.2% vs. 3.2%), fistula (3.1% vs. 1.1%), GI perforation (0.2%, 0.9%), proteinuria (0.7% vs. 1.4%), hemorrhage (0.2% vs. 0.9%), and myocardial infarction (0% vs. 1.1%)
- **Conclusion:**
  - → Longer BEV treatment for up to 30 months improves neither PFS nor OS; 15 months remain standard of care

Study: SOLO-1

- **Citation:** (Moore et al., 2018)
- **Highlight:** Upfront olaparib maintenance in BRCA+ patients
- **Design:**
  - 391 patients with newly diagnosed stage III or IV ovarian cancer, a mutation in BRCA1/2, and CR or PR after platinum-based CT randomized to 300 mg twice daily olaparib maintenance vs. placebo
- **Results:**
  - 388 patients with confirmed germline BRCA1/2 mutation; two with somatic mutations
  - Median follow-up: 41 months
  - Investigator assessed
    - HR for progression or death: 0.3 (CI = 0.23–0.41); p < 0.001
    - Rate of freedom from progression or death at 3 yrs: 60% vs. 27% (PFS in placebo group 13.8 months)
  - Assessed by independent review
    - HR for progression or death: 0.28 (CI = 0.20–0.39); p < 0.001
  - In sensitivity analysis: PSF about 36 months longer with olaparib
  - No new AEs
- **Conclusion:**
  - → Upfront olaparib maintenance therapy provided benefit with a 70% lower risk of disease progression or death than with placebo

Study: SOLO-1

- **Citation:** (DiSilvestro et al., 2020)
- **Highlight:** Subgroup analysis
- **Design:**
  - Investigator-assessed PFS subgroup analysis
- **Results:**
  - HR for disease progression or death
    - 0.31 and 0.37 in patients undergoing upfront or interval surgery

- 0.44 and 0.33 in patients with residual or no residual disease after surgery
- 0.34 and 0.31 in patients with CR or PR
- 0.41 and 0.2 in patients with BRCA1 or BRCA2
- **Conclusion:**
  - → In newly diagnosed ovarian cancer, substantial benefit from olaparib maintenance regardless of baseline surgery outcome, response to CT, and BRCA mutation type

Study: SOLO-1

- **Citation:** (Friedlander et al., 2021)
- **Highlight:** Patient-centered outcomes
- **Design:**
  - HRQOL was secondary endpoint and assessed by ovarian cancer Trial Outcome Index (TOI)
- **Results:**
  - No clinically meaningful change in TOI score at 24 months within or between the groups
  - Mean quality adjusted PFS: 29.8 vs. 17.6 months (olaparib vs. placebo; $p < 0.0001$)
  - Mean duration of time without significant symptoms of toxicity (TWiST): 33.2 vs. 20.2 months ($p < 0.0001$)
- **Conclusion:**
  - → Substantial PFS benefit with no detrimental effect on HRQOL supported by clinically meaningful quality adjusted PFS and TWiST

Study: PRIMA trial

- **Citation:** (Gonzalez-Martin et al., 2019)
- **Highlight:** Upfront niraparib maintenance
- **Design:**
  - 733 patients with newly diagnosed advanced ovarian cancer and response to platinum-based CT randomized in a 2:1 ratio to niraparib 300 or 200 mg po qd (if body weight <77 kg, or platelets <150 k) vs. placebo
- **Results:**
  - 50.9% with homologous recombination deficiency (defined as BRCA deleterious mutation, or score of ≥42 on MyChoice® test, Myriad Genetics, or both)
  - Homologous recombination deficient (HRD) group:
    - PFS: 21.9 vs. 10.4 months (niraparib vs. placebo) (HR 0.43 [CI = 0.31–0.59]; $p < 0.001$)
  - Overall population
    - PFS: 13.8 vs. 8.2 months (HR 0.62 [CI = 0.5–0.76]; $p < 0.001$)
    - At 24-month interim analysis OS: 84% vs. 77% (HR 0.7 [CI = 0.44–1.11])

- Subgroups (prespecified exploratory analyses)
  - HRD
    - BRCA mutation: PFS: 22.1 vs. 10.9 months
    - No BRCA mutation: PFS: 19.6 vs. 8.2 months
    - Homologous recombination proficient (HRP): PFS: 8.1 vs. 5.4 months
- Most common grade ≥3 AEs: anemia (31%), thrombocytopenia (28.7%), and neutropenia (12.8%)
- **Conclusion:**
  - → Niraparib prolongs PFS in patients with newly diagnosed advanced ovarian cancer and response to platinum-based treatment compared to placebo regardless of HR status

Study: PAOLA-1 trial

- **Citation:** (Ray-Coquard et al., 2019)
- **Highlight:** Olaparib + BEV in first-line maintenance
- **Design:**
  - 806 patients with newly diagnosed high-grade serous ovarian cancer and response to platinum-based CT plus BEV followed by BEV maintenance randomized 2:1 to olaparib 300 mg po bid vs. placebo for up to 24 months
- **Results:**
  - Median follow-up: 22.9 months
  - Overall
    - PFS: 22.1 vs. 16.6 months (olaparib + BEV vs. placebo + BEV; HR 0.59; CI = 0.49–0.72; p < 0.001)
  - HRD, including BRCA mutation
    - PFS: 37.2 vs. 17.7 months (HR 0.33; CI = 0.25–0.45)
  - HRD without BRCA mutation
    - PFS: 28.1 vs. 16.6 months (HR 0.43; CI = 0.28–0.66)
  - HRP or unknown status (419 patients)
    - PFS: 16.9 vs. 16.0 months (HR 0.92; CI = 0.72–1.17)
  - HRP (277 patients)
    - PFS: 16.6 vs. 16.2 months (HR 1.0; CI = 0.75–1.35)
  - No new safety signals
- **Conclusion:**
  - → Addition of olaparib to BEV provided significant PFS benefit in HRD tumors

2.1.5 Studies Addressing Neoadjuvant Therapy

Study: EORTC 55971 (European Organisation for Research and Treatment of Cancer)

- **Citation:** (Vergote et al., 2010)
- **Highlight:** NACT; non-inferiority trial

- **Design:**
    - 632 patients with stage IIIC or IV EOC randomized to primary debulking surgery (PDS) followed by at least 6 C platinum-based CT vs. 3 C neoadjuvant platinum-based CT followed by IDS, and then at least 3 C of platinum-based CT
    - Recommended CT
        - Paclitaxel 175 mg/m^2 over 3 hrs followed by carboplatin AUC 6 q 3 wks
        - Other regimens allowed, including cisplatin 75 mg/m^2 q 3 wks, or carboplatin AUC 5
    - IDS to be performed as soon as possible after hematologic recovery but within 6 wks after completion of third C; first C after surgery as soon as possible but no more than 6 wks
- **Results:**
    - Clinical stage IIIC: 76%; stage IV: 24%
    - Metastatic lesions >5 cm in 74.5% and >10 cm in 61.6%
    - Optimal cytoreduction in 41.6% in primary debulking and in 80.6% in IDS
    - At least 6 C: 82% vs. 86% (primary debulking vs. NACT)
    - AEs
        - Postoperative death: 2.5% vs. 0.7%
        - Hemorrhage ≥ grade 3: 7.6% vs. 4.1%
        - Infection ≥ grade 3: 8.1% vs. 1.7%
    - HR for progression (NACT compared to primary debulking): 1.01 (CI = 0.89–1.15)
    - HR for death: 0.98 (CI = 0.84–1.13); p = 0.01 for non-inferiority
    - Complete resection of all macroscopic disease (at primary or interval surgery) strongest independent variable in predicting OS
- **Conclusion:**
    - → NACT followed by IDS not inferior to primary debulking followed by CT for patients with bulky stage IIIC or IV disease
    - Complete resection remains the objective for PDS and IDS

Study: CHORUS trial (CHemotherapy OR Upfront Surgery)

- **Citation:** (Kehoe et al., 2015)
- **Highlight:** NACT; non-inferiority trial
- **Design:**
    - 550 patients with stage III or IV ovarian cancer randomized to primary surgery followed by 6 C platinum-based CT vs. 3 C of platinum-based primary CT followed by interval surgery and then followed by three more cycles CT
    - Each 3-weekly cycle: Carboplatin AUC 5 or 6 plus paclitaxel 175 mg/m^2, or alternative carboplatin combination or monotherapy
- **Results:**
    - Clinical stage III: 75%; stage IV: 25%
    - Median tumor size: >5 cm in 73% and >10 cm in 33%

- Optimal cytoreduction in 24% in primary surgery and 34% in NACT
  - Complete cytoreduction (no visible residual) 17% and 39%
- Single-agent carbo: 23%; carbo plus paclitaxel: 76%; carbo plus other agent: 1%
- 6 C carbo received: 82% vs. 79% (PDS vs. NACT)
- Grade 3 or 4 postoperative AEs: 24% vs. 14% (p = 0.0007)
- Deaths within 28 d: 6% vs. 1% (p = 0.001)
- Grade 3 or 4 CT-related toxic effect: 49% vs. 40% (p = 0.0654)
- Median OS: 22.6 vs. 24.1 months; HR for death 0.87 (CI = 0.72–1.05) in favor for primary CT
- **Conclusion:**
  - → In stage III or IV, primary CT is non-inferior to primary surgery; giving CT before surgery is acceptable standard in advanced ovarian cancer

Study: Pooled analysis of EORTC 55971 and CHORUS

- **Citation:** (Vergote et al., 2018)
- **Highlight:** OS benefit from NACT for stage IV ovarian cancer
- **Design:**
  - Pooled analysis of EORTC 55971 and CHORUS data to show non-inferiority in OS with NACT compared to upfront surgery
- **Results:**
  - 1,220 patients included
  - Median follow-up: 7.6 yrs
  - Median size of largest metastatic tumor: 8 cm
  - 5% with stage II–IIIB, 68% with stage IIIC, and 19% with stage IV
  - Median OS: 27.6 vs. 26.9 months (NACT vs. surgery)
  - Median OS EORTC vs. CHORUS: 30.2 vs. 23.6 months (HR 1.2 [CI = 1.06–1.36]; p = 0.004)
  - For stage IV, median OS: 24.3 vs. 21.2 months (HR 0.76 [CI = 0.58–1.00]; p = 0.048)
  - For stage IV, median PFS: 10.6 vs. 9.7 months (HR 0.77 [CI = 0.59–1.00]; p = 0.049)
- **Conclusion:**
  - → Long-term follow-up shows NACT results in similar OS in advanced EOC and better OS in stage IV EOC
  - NACT is a valuable treatment option for stages IIIC–IV, particularly with high tumor burden and poor performance status

Study: SCORPION trial

- **Citation:** (Fagotti et al., 2016)
- **Highlight:** Perioperative outcome data of NACT vs. primary debulking
- **Design:**
  - 110 patients with stage IIIC–IV ovarian cancer and peritoneal index (PI) of 8–12 randomized to PDS followed by adjuvant CT vs. NACT followed by IDS and CT

- Carboplatin/ paclitaxel-based CT in both arms
- Primary outcomes of superiority trial:
  - PFS and perioperative outcome
- **Results:**
  - No macroscopic residual disease: 45.5% vs. 57.7% (p = 0.206) (PDS vs. NACT)
  - Early grade 3 and 4 complications: 52.7% vs. 5.7% (p = 0.0001)
  - Most common grade 3: Pleural effusion: 30.9% vs. 1.9% (p = 0.0001)
  - Grade 4: Two reoperations and one septic multi-organ failure
  - Grade 5: Two deaths
  - Mean QoL scores ameliorate in both arms over time
    - Emotional functioning, cognitive functioning, nausea/vomiting, dyspnea, insomnia, and hair loss better in NACT
- **Conclusion:**
  - → Perioperative moderate/severe morbidity and QoL scores more favorable in NACT arm

Study: SCORPION trial

- **Citation:** (Fagotti et al., 2020)
- **Highlight:** PFS data of NACT vs. primary debulking
- **Design:**
  - 171 patients with stage IIIC–IV ovarian cancer and PI of 8–12 randomized to PDS followed by adjuvant CT vs. NACT followed by IDS and CT
- **Results:**
  - Median follow-up: 59 months
  - 84 patients underwent PDS and 87 underwent IDS
  - Complete gross resection: 47.6% vs. 77% (p = 0.001)
  - Major postoperative complications: 25.9% vs. 7.6% (p = 0.0001)
  - Deaths: 7 vs. 0 deaths (p = 0.006)
  - PFS: 15 vs. 14 months (HR 1.05 [CI = 0.77–1.44]; p = 0.73) (PDS vs. NACT)
  - OS: 41 vs. 43 months (HR 1.05; CI = 0.77–1.44; p = 0.56)
- **Conclusion:**
  - → NACT and PDS with the same efficacy but different toxicity profile

2.1.6 Studies Addressing Prediction of Debulking

Study: Suidan study

- **Citation:** (Suidan et al., 2014)
- **Highlight:** CT- and CA-125-based prediction
- **Design:**
  - To assess ability of preoperative CT scan and serum CA-125 to predict suboptimal (>1 cm) primary cytoreduction: 669 patients prospectively enrolled; 350 eligible

- **Results:**
  - Optimal debulking rate: 75%
  - On multivariate analysis, three clinical and six radiological criteria associated with suboptimal debulking
    - Age ≥60 (p = 0.01)
    - CA-125 ≥500 U/mL (p < 0.001)
    - American Society of Anesthesiologists (ASA) class 3–4 (p < 0.001)
    - Suprarenal retroperitoneal LNs >1 cm (p < 0.001)
    - Diffuse small bowel adhesions/thickening (p < 0.001)
    - Lesions >1 cm in small bowel mesentery (p = 0.03)
    - Lesions >1 cm in root of superior mesenteric artery (p = 0.003)
    - Lesions >1 cm in perisplenic area (p < 0.001)
    - Lesions >1 cm in lesser sac (p < 0.001)
  - Predictive value score assigned to each criterion
    - Suboptimal debulking rates with total score of 0, 1–2, 3–4, 5–6, 7–8, ≥9 were 5%, 10%, 17%, 34%, 52%, and 74%
    - Prognostic model with predictive accuracy of 0.758
- **Conclusion:**
  - → Definition of nine criteria associated with suboptimal cytoreduction and development of predictive model, in which suboptimal rate is directly proportional to predictive value score

Study: Fagotti score

- **Citation:** (Fagotti et al., 2008)
- **Highlight:** Laparoscopy-based score
- **Design:**
  - To validate a laparoscopy-based model to predict optimal cytoreduction
  - Prospective study: 113 patients with advanced ovarian cancer: Presence of omental cake, peritoneal and diaphragmatic extensive carcinomatosis, mesenteric retraction, bowel or stomach infiltration, spleen, and/or liver superficial metastasis investigated by LSC
  - All women underwent LSC and then exlap; same surgical team
  - Trial included cases of IDS with suboptimal response after NACT
  - Trial excluded large masses reaching xiphoid, occupying entire abdominal cavity and/or infiltrating abdominal wall
  - Total predictive index value = PIV (sum of all scores)
- **Results:**
  - Accuracy: 77.3–100% (LSC compared to exlap)
    - Least accurate: Bowel infiltration 77.3% and superficial liver metastasis 88.7%; all other parameters ≥95% accurate
  - PIV ≥8: Probability of optimal resection equals 0, and rate of unnecessary exlap is 40.5%
- **Conclusion:**
  - → Proposed LSC model reliable and flexible tool to predict optimal cytoreduction

Study: Petrillo study

- **Citation:** (Petrillo et al., 2015)
- **Highlight:** LSC-based score
- **Design:**
  - To develop LSC-based model to predict incomplete cytoreduction (presence of macroscopic disease >0 cm)
  - Prospective study of 234 patients with newly diagnosed advanced EOC
  - Staging LSC evaluated omental cake, extensive peritoneal carcinomatosis, confluent diaphragmatic carcinomatosis, bowel infiltration, stomach and/or spleen and/or lesser omentum infiltration, and superficial liver metastases
  - Staging LSC followed by PDS
- **Results:**
  - Parameters with specificity ≥75%, PPV ≥50%, NPV ≥50% received 1 point; one additional point if accuracy ≥60% in predicting complete cytoreduction
  - High overall agreement ranging from 74.7% for omental cake to 94.8% for stomach infiltration
  - PIV ≥10: Chance of achieving complete cytoreduction was 0; risk of unnecessary laparotomy 33.2%
- **Conclusion:**
  - → Staging LSC accurate tool in predicting complete debulking, improved performance, with lower rate of inappropriate exlaps at cutoff value of 10

2.1.7 Studies Addressing Time Point of Treatment for Recurrence

Study: MRC OV05/EORTC 55955

- **Citation:** (Rustin et al., 2010)
- **Highlight:** Treatment of serum vs. clinical recurrence
- **Design:**
  - Serum CA-125 often rises several months before clinical relapse; here, to assess benefits of early treatment (on basis of increased CA-125) vs. delayed treatment (on basis of clinical recurrence)
  - 1,442 patients with ovarian cancer in complete remission after first-line platinum-based CT and normal CA-125 enrolled; clinical exams and CA-125 q 3 months; patients and investigators masked to CA-125 results (monitored by coordinating centers)
  - If CA-125 >2 ULN patients randomized to early or delayed CT; if not randomized to immediate treatment, continued to be monitor and treatment when clinical relapse; in total, 529 patients randomized
- **Results:**
  - Median follow-up: 56.9 months

- No difference in median OS: 25.7 vs. 27.1 months (early vs. delayed) (HR 0.98 [CI = 0.8–1.2]; p = 0.85)
- **Conclusion:**
  - → No e/o survival benefit with early treatment of relapse based on raised CA-125; therefore, value of routine CA-125 in follow-up in patients who attain CR after first-line CT not proven

2.1.8 Studies Addressing Treatment of Recurrent Ovarian Cancer, Platinum Sensitive

2.1.8.1 Chemotherapy and Targeted Therapy

Study: ICON4/AGO-OVAR-2.2 trial

- **Citation:** (Parmar et al., 2003)
- **Highlight:** Addition of Taxol to carbo for recurrent platinum-sensitive EOC
- **Design:**
  - 802 patients with platinum-sensitive recurrent ovarian cancer randomized to paclitaxel plus platinum vs. conventional platinum-based CT
  - Conventional CT:
    - Single-agent carboplatin (71%)
    - Cyclophosphamide, doxorubicin, and cisplatin CAP (17%)
    - Switched between single-agent cisplatin and carboplatin (4%)
    - Cisplatin and doxorubicin (3%)
    - Single-agent cisplatin (2%)
- **Results:**
  - At least 6 C: 78% vs. 67% (carbo/Taxol vs. conventional)
  - Median follow-up: 42 months
  - 1-yr PFS: 50 vs. 40% (HR for progression 0.76 [CI = 0.66–0.89]; p = 0.0004)
  - Median PFS: 13 vs. 10 months
  - 2-yr OS: 57 vs. 50% (HR for death: 0.82 [CI = 0.69–0.97]; p = 0.02)
  - Median OS: 29 vs. 24 months
- **Conclusion:**
  - → Paclitaxel plus platinum CT regimen improves PFS and OS among patients with relapsed platinum-sensitive ovarian cancer compared with conventional platinum-based CT

Study: Pfisterer study

- **Citation:** (Pfisterer et al., 2006)
- **Highlight:** Carbo/Gem, possible alternative to carbo in recurrent platinum-sensitive EOC
- **Background:**
  - Most patients with advanced ovarian cancer develop recurrence; if recur at least 6 months after initial therapy, paclitaxel and platinum showed

modest survival advantage over platinum without paclitaxel; however, relevant neurotoxicity resulting in discontinuation; need for alternative regimens without neurotoxicity

- **Design:**
  - 356 patients with platinum-sensitive recurrent ovarian cancer randomized to gemcitabine 1,000 mg/m^2 on days 1 and 8 plus carboplatin AUC 4 on day 1 q 3 wks × 6 C vs. single-agent carboplatin AUC 5 q 3 wks × 6 C
- **Results:**
  - Median follow-up: 17 months
  - Myelosuppression more common, but febrile neutropenia or infections uncommon
  - No significant difference in QoL
  - Median PFS: 8.6 vs. 5.8 months (gemcitabine plus carbo vs. carbo) (HR 0.72; p = 0.0031)
  - Response rate: 47.2% vs. 30.9% (p = 0.0016)
  - HR for OS: 0.96 (CI = 0.75–1.23)
- **Conclusion:**
  - → Gemcitabine plus carbo improves PFS and response rates without worsening QoL in platinum-sensitive recurrent ovarian cancer

Study: OCEANS trial

- **Citation:** (Aghajanian et al., 2012)
- **Highlight:** Carbo/gem +/– BEV
- **Design:**
  - 484 patients with platinum-sensitive recurrent ovarian cancer randomized to gemcitabine 1,000 mg/m^2 on days 1 and 8 and carboplatin AUC 4 on day 1 q 3 wks × 6(–10) C vs. gemcitabine 1,000 mg/m^2 on days 1 and 8 and carboplatin AUC 4 on day 1 plus BEV 15 mg/kg on day 1 q 3 wks × 6(–10) C, followed by BEV as maintenance
- **Results:**
  - No new safety concerns noted
    - HTN ≥ grade 3: 17.4% vs. <1% (BEV vs. placebo)
    - Proteinuria: 8.5% vs. <1%
    - Rates of neutropenia and febrile neutropenia similar
    - 2 GI perforations after treatment discontinuation
  - ORR: 78.5% vs. 57.4% (p < 0.0001)
  - DOR: 10.4 vs. 7.4 months
  - Median PFS: 12.4 vs. 8.4 months (p < 0.0001)
- **Conclusion:**
  - → GC plus BEV followed by BEV improved PFS compared to GC in platinum-sensitive recurrent ovarian cancer

Study: OCEANS trial

- **Citation:** (Aghajanian et al., 2015)
- **Highlight:** Long-term follow-up

- **Results:**
  - Median follow-up: 58.2 months
  - Median OS: 33.6 vs. 32.9 months (p = 0.65)
  - No new safety concerns
- **Conclusion:**
  - → No difference in OS

Study: CALYPSO trial

- **Citation:** (Pujade-Lauraine et al., 2010)
- **Highlight:** Carbo/Taxol vs. carbo/doxil
- **Design:**
  - Non-inferiority trial: 976 patients with platinum-sensitive recurrent ovarian cancer randomized to carboplatin AUC 5 plus paclitaxel 175 mg/m^2 q 3 wks × at least 6 C (CP) vs. carboplatin AUC 5 plus PLD 30 mg/m^2 q 4 wks × at least 6 C
- **Results:**
  - Toxicities (PLD vs. CP)
    - Severe non-hematologic toxicity: 28.4% vs. 36.8% (p < 0.01), leading to early discontinuation 6% vs. 15% (p < 0.001)
    - Alopecia ≥ grade 2: 7% vs. 83.6%
    - Hypersensitivity reaction: 5.6% vs. 18.8%
    - Sensory neuropathy: 4.9% vs. 26.9%
    - Hand–foot syndrome grade 2 or 3: 12% vs. 2.2%
    - Nausea: 35.2% vs 24.2%
    - Mucositis grade 2 or 3: 13.9% vs. 7%
  - Median follow-up: 22 months
  - Median PFS: 11.3 vs. 9.4 months (PLD vs. CP) (p = 0.005)
- **Conclusion:**
  - → Demonstrated superiority in PFS and therapeutic index of carbo/PLD over standard carbo/paclitaxel

Study: CALYPSO trial

- **Citation:** (Wagner et al., 2012)
- **Highlight:** Long-term follow-up
- **Results:**
  - Median follow-up: 49 months
  - Median OS: 30.7 vs. 33.0 months (PLD vs. CP)
  - No difference in predetermined subgroups
    - Age, body mass index (BMI), treatment-free interval, measurable disease, number of prior lines of CT, and performance status
  - Post-study crossover more frequently to PLD (p < 0.001)
- **Conclusion:**
  - → Carbo/PLD delayed progression and has similar OS compared to CP–paclitaxel in platinum-sensitive recurrent ovarian cancer

Study: Gordon trial

- **Citation:** (Gordon et al., 2001)
- **Highlight:** Doxil vs. topotecan
- **Design:**
  - 474 patients with ovarian cancer that recurred or did not respond to first-line platinum-based CT randomized to PLD 50 mg/m² over 1 hr q 4 wks vs. topotecan 1.5 mg/m² for 5 consecutive days q 3 wks
  - Stratified prospectively by platinum sensitivity and bulky disease
  - 46–47% platinum-sensitive in each group
- **Results:**
  - Severe hematologic toxicity more common with topotecan
  - PFS similar (p = 0.095)
  - Response rates: 19.7% vs. 17.0% (PLD vs. topotecan)
  - Median OS: 60 vs. 56.7 weeks
  - In platinum sensitive
    - Median PFS: 28.9 vs. 23.3 weeks (p = 0.037)
    - Median OS: 108 vs. 71.1 weeks (p = 0.008)
  - In platinum resistant
    - Nonsignificant OS trend in favor of topotecan (p = 0.455)
  - No difference in outcome for bulky disease (>5 cm)
- **Conclusion:**
  - → Comparable efficacy, favorable safety profile, and convenient dosing support PLD as treatment option

Study: Pfisterer trial

- **Citation:** (Pfisterer et al., 2020)
- **Highlight:** Carbo/doxil + BEV
- **Design:**
  - 682 patients with first recurrence of platinum-sensitive ovarian cancer randomized to six cycles of BEV 15 mg/kg plus carboplatin AUC 4 plus gemcitabine 1,000 mg/m² on days 1 and 8 q 3 wks (standard) vs. six cycles of BEV 10 mg/kg on days 1 and 15 plus carboplatin AUC 5 plus PLD 30 mg/m² q 4 wks (experimental); both followed by maintenance BEV 15 mg/kg q 3 wks
- **Results:**
  - Median PFS: 13.3 vs. 11.6 months (HR 0.81; CI = 0.68–0.96; p = 0.012) (exp vs. std)
  - ≥Grade 3 AEs: hypertension (27% vs. 20%) and neutropenia (12% vs. 22%)
- **Conclusion:**
  - → Carbo + PLD + BEV is a new standard treatment option for platinum-eligible recurrent ovarian cancer.

Study: Study 19

- **Citation:** (Ledermann et al., 2012)
- **Highlight:** Olaparib maintenance
- **Design:**
  - Olaparib = PARP 1/2 inhibitor
  - Phase II trial: 265 patients with recurrent platinum-sensitive high-grade serous ovarian cancer, ≥2 prior platinum-based chemotherapies, and at least PR to most recent platinum-based CT randomized to olaparib 400 mg bid po vs. placebo
  - In recurrent platinum-sensitive high-grade serous ovarian cancers, tumor cells highly enriched for homologous-recombination deficiency
  - Primary endpoint: PFS
  - Secondary endpoint: OS (hence not powered to assess statistical significance in OS difference)
  - Stratified by interval between disease progression and completion of their penultimate platinum-based regimen (6–12 and >12 months), objective response rate to most recent regimen (CR vs. PR), and ancestry (Jewish vs. non-Jewish) to help balance BRCA 1/2 germline mutation
- **Results:**
  - AEs (olaparib vs. placebo)
    - Nausea: 68% vs. 35%
    - Fatigue: 49% vs. 38%
    - Vomiting: 32% vs. 14%
    - Anemia: 17% vs. 5%
    - Majority grade 1 or 2
  - Median PFS: 8.4 vs. 4.8 months (HR = 0.35 [CI = 0.25–0.49]; $p < 0.001$)
    - PFS longer regardless of subgroup
  - Interim analysis of OS (38% maturity): HR 0.94 (CI = 0.63–1.39); $p = 0.75$
- **Conclusion:**
  - → Olaparib as maintenance improved PFS in platinum-sensitive high-grade serous ovarian cancer

Study: Study 19

- **Citation:** (Ledermann et al., 2014)
- **Highlight:** Olaparib maintenance; preplanned retrospective analysis of outcomes by BRCA status
- **Design:**
  - Hypothesis: Olaparib most likely benefits patients with BRCA mutation
  - BRCA status known: 131/136 (96%) in olaparib group and 123/129 (95%) in placebo group
    - 74 (56%) vs. 62 (50%) with deleterious or suspected deleterious germline or tumor BRCA mutation

- **Results:**
  - Median PFS
    - In BRCAm: 11.2 vs. 4.3 months (HR 0.18 [CI = 0.1–0.31]; p < 0.0001)
    - In BRCAwt: 7.4 vs. 5.5 months (HR 0.54 [CI = 0.34–0.85]; p = 0.0075)
  - Median OS (58% maturity): HR 0.88 (CI = 0.64–1.21); p = 0.44
    - BRCAm: HR 0.73 (CI = 0.45–1.17); p = 0.19
    - BRCAwt: HR 0.99 (CI = 0.63–1.55); p = 0.96
- **Conclusion:**
  - → Results support hypothesis that BRCAm recurrent platinum-sensitive serous EOC has greatest benefit from olaparib

Study: Study 19

- **Citation:** (Ledermann et al., 2016)
- **Highlight:** Olaparib maintenance; updated analysis
- **Results:**
  - Median OS for all patients: 29.8 vs. 27.8 months (p = 0.025) (predefined significance p < 0.0095)
    - Median OS for BRCAm patients: 34.9 vs. 30.2 months (p = 0.025) (predefined significance p < 0.0095)
    - Median OS for BRCAwt patients: 24.6 vs 26.6 months
  - 11/74 patients (15%) with BRCAm received maintenance therapy for ≥5 yrs
- **Conclusion:**
  - → Improvement in OS did not reach statistical significance
  - No new safety signals after long-term exposure
  - 'These data support both long-term clinical benefit and tolerability of maintenance olaparib in patients with BRCAm recurrent platinum-sensitive serous ovarian cancer'.

Study: Study 42

- **Citation:** (Domchek et al., 2016)
- **Highlight:** Olaparib monotherapy of relapsed ovarian cancer in gBRCAm regardless of platinum sensitivity
- **Design:**
  - Phase II study enrolled 193 patients; 154/193 (80%) had received ≥3 lines
- **Results:**
  - Overall ORR: 34% (CI: 26–42%)
  - Median DoR: 7.9 months
  - ORR in platinum resistant: 30%
  - Median DoR: 8.2 (platinum sensitive) and 8.0 (platinum resistant)
- **Conclusion:**
  - → Following ≥3 lines, olaparib 400 mg bid with notable antitumor activity in patients with gBRCAm ovarian cancer regardless of platinum sensitivity

Study: NOVA trial

- **Citation:** (Mirza et al., 2016)
- **Highlight:** Niraparib maintenance
- **Design:**
  - Niraparib = PARP 1/2 inhibitor
  - 553 patients with recurrent platinum-sensitive high-grade serous ovarian cancer with ≥2 prior chemotherapies stratified by the presence or absence of germline mutation gBRCA and non-gBRCA and type of non-gBRCA mutation and 2:1 randomized to niraparib 300 mg qd po vs. placebo
  - MyChoice HRD (homologous recombination deficiency) test used to define non-gBRCA cohort
    - In MyChoice, LOH, telomeric allelic imbalance, and large-scale state transitions are used to assess genomic instability
    - Non-gBRCA classified as
      - HRD positive
        - HRD positive/sBRCAmut (with somatic BRCA mutation)
        - HRD positive/BRCAwt (i.e., with other dysregulations in homologous recombination DNA repair)
      - HRD negative
- **Results:**
  - 203/553 with gBRCAmut; 350/553 with non-gBRCAmut
  - Median PFS
    - gBRCA group: 21 vs. 5.5 months (p < 0.001) (niraparib vs. placebo)
    - Non-gBRCA group, overall: 9.3 vs. 3.9 months (p < 0.001)
      - Non-gBRCAmut HRD positive: 12.9 vs. 3.8 months (p < 0.001)
        - HRD positive/BRCAwt: 9.3 vs. 3.7 months (p < 0.001)
        - HRD positive/sBRCAmut: 20.9 vs. 11 months (p = 0.02)
      - Non-gBRCAmut HRD negative: 6.9 vs. 3.8 months (p = 0.02)
  - Grade 3 or 4 AEs
    - Thrombocytopenia: 33.8% vs. 0.6% (Del Campo et al., 2019)
    - Anemia: 25.3% vs. 0%
    - Neutropenia: 19.6% vs. 1.7%
    - Managed with dose modifications
- **Conclusion:**
  - → Among patients with recurrent platinum-sensitive ovarian cancer, median PFS significantly longer regardless of presence or absence of gBRCA mutation or HRD status, with moderate bone marrow toxicity

Study: NOVA trial

- **Citation:** (Del Campo et al., 2019)
- **Highlight:** Niraparib maintenance after PR
- **Results:**
  - In gBRCA cohort, patients with PR had longer PFS with niraparib compared to placebo (HR 0.24 [CI = 0.13–0.44]; p < 0.0001)

- In non-gBRCA cohort, patients with PR had longer PFS with niraparib compared to placebo (HR 0.35 [CI = 0.23–0.53]; p < 0.0001)
- **Conclusion:**
  - → Clinical benefit from niraparib maintenance regardless of response to last platinum-based therapy

Study: SOLO2/ENGOT-Ov21

- **Citation:** (Pujade-Lauraine et al., 2017)
- **Highlight:** Olaparib maintenance in gBRCAmut
- **Design:**
  - Double-blind phase III trial: 295 patients with germline BRCA1/2 mutation and recurrent platinum-sensitive high-grade serous ovarian cancer and ≥2 prior chemotherapies randomized 2:1 to olaparib 300 mg qd po vs. placebo
  - Stratified by interval between disease progression and completion of their penultimate platinum-based regimen (6–12 and >12 months), objective response rate to most recent regimen (CR vs. PR)
- **Results:**
  - Most common ≥ grade 3 AEs (olaparib vs. placebo)
    - Anemia: 19% vs. 2%
    - Fatigue: 4% vs. 2%
    - Neutropenia: 5% vs. 4%
  - Median PFS: 19.1 vs. 5.5 months (p < 0.0001)
- **Conclusion:**
  - → Olaparib maintenance with improvement in PFS and no detrimental effect on QoL in recurrent platinum-sensitive high-grade serous ovarian cancer and BRCA1/2 mutation; apart from anemia, mainly low-grade toxicities

Study: SOLO2/ENGOT-Ov21

- **Citation:** (Poveda et al., 2021)
- **Highlight:** Final analysis
- **Results:**
  - Median follow-up: 66 months
  - Most common ≥ grade 3 AEs (olaparib vs. placebo)
    - Anemia: 21% vs. 2%
    - MDS/AML: 8% vs. 4% (9/16 vs. 4/4 developed after safety follow-up period)
  - Median OS: 51.7 vs. 38.8 months (HR 74 [CI = 0.54–1.0]; p = 0.054), unadjusted for the 38% in the placebo group who received subsequent PARP inhibitor treatment
- **Conclusion:**
  - → Olaparib provided median OS benefit of 12.9 months in patients with platinum-sensitive, relapsed ovarian cancer, and BRCA1/2 mutation

Study: ARIEL 2 Part 1

- **Citation:** (Swisher et al., 2017)
- **Highlight:** LOH high used to predict response to rucaparib treatment in BRCAwt
- **Design:**
  - Phase II: 206 patients with recurrent platinum-sensitive high-grade (serous and endometrioid) ovarian cancer, measurable disease, and at least one prior platinum-based CT received rucaparib 600 mg bid qd po
  - 192 patients classified into predefined homologous recombination deficiency subgroups
    - BRCAm (somatic or germline): (n = 40)
    - Genome-wide LOH in the tumor: LOH high (n = 82)
    - LOH low: (n = 70)
- **Results:**
  - Most common ≥ grade 3 AEs
    - Anemia (22%)
    - Elevated LFTs (12%)
  - Median PFS: 12.8 and 5.7 vs. 5.2 months (BRCAm [p < 0.0001] and LOH high [p = 0.011] vs. LOH low)
- **Conclusion:**
  - → Assessment of tumor LOH can be used to identify patients with BRCAwt platinum-sensitive ovarian cancer who might benefit from rucaparib treatment

Study: ARIEL 3

- **Citation:** (Coleman et al., 2017b)
- **Highlight:** Rucaparib maintenance
- **Design:**
  - 564 patients with recurrent platinum-sensitive ovarian cancer after ≥2 prior platinum-based CT regimens, at least PR to last CT and normal CA-125 randomized to rucaparib 600 mg bid po vs. placebo
  - Stratified by homologous recombination repair gene mutation status, PFS after penultimate platinum-based regimen; best response to most recent platinum-based regimen
- **Results:**
  - Groups
    - gBRCAmut (130) or sBRCAmut (56)
    - BRCAwt HRD positive (i.e., LOH high [158])
    - BRCAwt and LOH low or indeterminate (210)
  - ≥ Grade 3 AEs: 56% vs. 15% (rucaparib vs. placebo)
    - Anemia: 19% vs. 1%
    - Elevated LFTs: 10% vs. none
  - Median PFS with BRCA mutation (germline or somatic): 16.6 vs. 5.4 months (p < 0.0001)

- Median PFS with HRD carcinoma (includes gBRCAm, sBRCAm, and BRCAwt LOH high): 13.6 vs. 5.4 months (p < 0.0001)
- In intention-to-treat population (includes all): 10.8 vs. 5.4 months (p < 0.0001)
- **Conclusion:**
  - → Across all primary analysis groups, rucaparib maintenance therapy significantly improved PFS in platinum-sensitive ovarian cancer; further evidence that PARPi in maintenance setting is new standard

Study: ARIEL 4

- **Citation:** (Kristeleit et al., 2022)
- **Highlight:** Rucaparib treatment
- **Design:**
  - 349 patients with recurrent BRCA-mutated ovarian cancers with ≥2 prior lines 2:1 randomized to 600 mg BID rucaparib po vs. CT (platinum based for platinum-sensitive disease or weekly paclitaxel for platinum-resistant disease)
- **Results:**
  - Median follow-up: 25.0 months
  - 50% platinum-resistant in efficacy population
  - In efficacy population (all randomly assigned patients with deleterious BRCA mutations without reversion mutation)
    - Median PFS: 7.4 vs. 5.7 months (HR 0.64 [CI: 0.49–0.84]; p = 0.001) (rucaparib vs. CT)
      - PFS in platinum resistant: 6.4 vs. 6.7 months
      - PFS in partially platinum-resistant (recurrence 6–12 months after last platinum-based CT): 8.0 vs. 5.5 months
      - PFS in platinum sensitive: 12.9 vs. 9.6 months
  - Serious AEs: 27% vs. 12%
- **Conclusion:**
  - → This study supports rucaparib as alternative treatment option to CT with relapsed BRCA-mutated ovarian cancer

Study: QUADRA

- **Citation**: (Moore et al., 2019)
- **Highlight:** Niraparib monotherapy for late-line treatment
- **Design:**
  - Phase II trial: 463 patients with recurrent high-grade serous ovarian cancer on ≥3 prior chemotherapies (including prior PARPi) received 300 mg niraparib po qd
- **Results:**
  - Median of four prior lines
    - 37 patients with prior PARP inhibitor treatment

- HRD status
  - Positive: 189/419 (PARP inhibitor naïve)
    - 63 BRCAm
      - 18 platinum sensitive
      - 37 platinum resistant
      - 8 unknown
    - 126 non-BRCAm
      - 29 platinum sensitive in fourth or fifth line
      - 6 platinum sensitive in ≥ sixth line
      - 83 platinum resistant
      - 8 unknown
  - Negative: 186/419
    - 41 platinum sensitive
    - 137 platinum resistant or refractory
    - 8 unknown
  - Unknown: 44/419
    - 11 platinum sensitive
    - 32 platinum resistant or refractory
    - 1 unknown
- Median follow-up: 12.2 months
- 151/463 (33%) patients resistant to last platinum treatment
- 161/ 463 (35%) refractory
- In primary efficacy population (three or four prior lines, HRD positive, platinum sensitive, and PARP inhibitor naïve)
  - ORR: 13/47 (28%)
  - Median PFS: 5.5 months
  - Median DoR: 9.2 months
  - DCR: 32/47 (68%)
- In response-evaluable patients
  - ORR: 38/387 (10%)
- In modified per-protocol population
  - ORR: 38/456 (8%)
- Prespecified exploratory analyses
  - BRCAm and platinum sensitive, ORR: 7/18 (39%)
  - BRCAm and platinum resistant, ORR: 10/37 (27%)
  - HRDpos and platinum sensitive, ORR: 14/53 (26%)
  - HRDpos and platinum resistant, ORR: 12/120 (10%)
- Most common ≥ grade 3 AEs
  - Anemia: 24%
  - Thrombocytopenia: 21%
- One treatment-related death: gastric hemorrhage
- **Conclusion:**
  - → Clinically relevant activity of niraparib in heavily pretreated ovarian cancer, especially in HRD-positive (BRCA + and wild type) platinum-sensitive disease

Study: OReO trial (NCT03106987), ongoing

- **Citation**: Abstract, presented at ESMO (Pujade-Lauraine et al., 2021)
- **Highlight:** PARP after PARP
- **Design:**
  - 220 patients with recurrent platinum-sensitive ovarian cancer and one line of prior PARP inhibitor randomized 2:1 to olaparib maintenance 300 (or 250) mg BID, stratified by prior BEV and number of prior platinum-based CT lines
- **Results:**
  - Heavily pretreated: 93% (in BRCAm) and 86% (in non-BRCAm) with ≥3 prior lines
  - BRCAm
    - PFS: 4.3 vs. 2.8 months
  - Non-BRCAm
    - PFS: 5.3 vs. 2.8 months
  - Grade ≥3 AEs in 15% vs. 5% (BRCAm) and 21% vs. 8% (non-BRCAm)
- **Conclusion:**
  - → First trial with data on PARPi rechallenge; maintenance olaparib provided improvement in PFS

Study: GOG 213

- **Citation:** (Coleman et al., 2017a)
- **Highlight:** Addition of BEV for recurrent platinum-sensitive EOC
- **Design:**
  - Bifactorial phase III trial with BEV objective and secondary cytoreduction objective; here, BEV objective reported
  - 674 patients with platinum-sensitive recurrent ovarian cancer and CR to primary treatment randomized to paclitaxel 175 mg/m^2 and carboplatin AUC 5 q 3 wks vs. paclitaxel 175 mg/m^2 and carboplatin AUC 5 plus BEV 15 mg/kg q 3 wks and continued as maintenance q 3 wks
  - Patients who participated in both, BEV objective and surgical objective (which is ongoing), were randomized 1:1:1:1 to receive either CT with or without surgery
  - Randomization for BEV objective stratified by treatment-free interval and participation in surgical objective
- **Results:**
  - Median number of BEV cycles: 16
  - Median follow-up: 49.6 months
  - At least one grade 3 or greater AEs: 317/325 (96%) in BEV group vs. 282/332 (86%) in CT group
    - HTN: 12% vs. 1%
    - Fatigue: 8% vs. 2%
    - Proteinuria: 8% vs. 0%
    - Treatment-related deaths: 3% vs. 1%

- Median PFS: 13.8 vs 10.4 months (p < 0.0001) (BEV vs. standard)
  - Consistent across subgroups: Participation in surgical objective, platinum-free interval, and previous BEV treatment
- Median OS: 42.2 vs. 37.7 (p = 0.056)
  - Identified incorrect treatment-free interval stratification for 45 patients (7%) (adjusted HR 0.823; p = 0.0447)
- **Conclusion:**
  - → Addition of BEV to standard CT followed by maintenance improved median OS in platinum-sensitive recurrent ovarian cancer

Study: MITO16B/MaNGO OV2B/ENGOT OV17

- **Citation:** (Pignata et al., 2021)
- **Highlight:** BEV + platinum after BEV + platinum
- **Design:**
  - 406 patients with recurrent platinum-sensitive ovarian cancer who had received BEV during first line randomized to platinum doublets (carboplatin AUC 5/ paclitaxel 175 mg/m^2 q 21 d; carboplatin AUC 4/ gemcitabine 1,000 mg/m^2 on days 1 and 8 q 21 d; carboplatin AUC 5/ PLD 30 mg/m^2 q 28 d) without vs. with BEV 15 mg/kg q 3 wks and 10 mg/ kg q 2 wks for carboplatin plus PLD concomitant and as maintenance 15 mg/kg q 3 wks
- **Results:**
  - 72% had progressed ≥12 months after last platinum, and 72% had progressed after completion of first-line BEV maintenance
  - ORR: 49.7% vs. 69.2% (p = 0.001) (without vs. with BEV)
    - CR: 11.2% vs. 23.8%
    - PR: 38.5% vs. 45.5%
  - Median PFS: 8.8 vs. 11.8 months (HR 0.51 [CI = 0.41–0.64]; p < 0.001)
  - Median OS: 27.1 vs. 26.7 months
  - AEs
    - Grade ≥3 HTN: 10% vs. 29%
    - Grade ≥3 proteinuria: 0% vs. 4%
- **Conclusion:**
  - → Rechallenge with BEV in combination with platinum doublets associated with prolonged PFS; no unexpected toxicity

Study: AVANOVA trial

- **Citation:** (Mirza et al., 2019)
- **Highlight:** Treatment with niraparib plus BEV
- **Design:**
  - In randomized phase II trial, 97 patients with recurrent platinum-sensitive ovarian cancer, previous BEV, and PARP inhibitor maintenance permitted, randomized to 300 mg niraparib po qd plus 15 mg/kg BEV iv q 3 wks vs. single-agent 300 mg niraparib qd po

- **Results:**
  - Median follow-up: 16.9 months
  - Median PFS: 11.9 vs. 5.5 months (HR 0.35 [CI = 0.21–0.57]; p < 0.0001) (niraparib + BEV vs. niraparib)
  - ≥ Grade 3 AEs: 65% vs. 45%
    - Anemia (15% vs. 18%), thrombocytopenia (10% vs. 12%), and hypertension (21% vs. 0%)
- **Conclusion:**
  - → Efficacy of combination in recurrent platinum-sensitive ovarian cancer warrants further evaluation

2.1.8.2 Secondary Debulking Surgery

Study: Salani study

- **Citation:** (Salani et al., 2007)
- **Highlight:** Secondary debulking
- **Design:**
  - Retrospective study: 55 patients undergoing secondary surgical cytoreduction for recurrent EOC
    - Inclusion criteria
      - CR to primary treatment
      - ≥12 months between initial diagnosis and recurrence
      - ≤5 recurrence sites on preoperative imaging
- **Results:**
  - In 41/55 (74.5%): Complete cytoreduction
  - On multivariate analysis, independent predictors:
    - Interval to recurrence: ≥18 months (p < 0.01)
    - Number of radiographic recurrence sites: Median survival 50 months for one to two sites vs. 12 months for three to five sites (p < 0.03)
    - Residual disease: Median survival 50 months for no macroscopic disease vs. 7.2 months for macroscopic residual disease (p < 0.01)
  - Age, tumor grade, histology, CA-125, ascites, and tumor size not associated significantly with survival
- **Conclusion:**
  - → These data support the definition of localized recurrent ovarian cancer as one or two radiographic sites; in this population, an interval ≥18 months and complete cytoreduction associated with median post-recurrence survival of 50 months

Study: AGO DESKTOP OVAR I

- **Citation:** (Harter et al., 2006)
- **Highlight:** AGO score for secondary debulking developed based on retrospective data

- **Design:**
  - Descriptive Evaluation of preoperative Selection Kriteria for Operability in recurrent Ovarian cancer to form criteria for selecting patients who might benefit from surgery in relapsed ovarian cancer
  - Retrospective study: 276 patients included
- **Results:**
  - Complete resection associated with significantly longer survival 45.2 vs. 19.7 months (p < 0.0001)
  - Associated with complete resection:
    - Performance status (ECOG score 0 vs. >0; p = 0.001)
    - Stage at initial diagnosis (stage I/II vs. III/IV; p = 0.036)
    - Residual tumor at primary surgery (none vs. present; p < 0.001)
    - Absence of ascites >500 mL (p < 0.001)
    - Combination of performance status, early stage initially or no residual tumor at first surgery, and absence of ascites predicted complete resection in 79%
- **Conclusion:**
  - → Only complete resection associated with prolonged survival in recurrent cancer; criteria to be verified in prospective trial

Study: AGO DESKTOP OVAR II

- **Citation:** (Harter et al., 2011)
- **Highlight:** Prospective validation of AGO score
- **Design:**
  - Prospective study: 516 patients with platinum-sensitive first or second relapse enrolled
  - Resectability assumed if three factors present
    - Complete resection at first surgery
    - Good performance status
    - Absence of ascites
- **Results:**
  - 261/516 (51%) classified score positive
  - 126 patients with positive score and first relapse were operated on; rate of complete resection 76%
  - Complication rates moderate; perioperative mortality 0.8%
- **Conclusion:**
  - → Score is first prospectively validated instrument to predict surgical outcome in recurrent ovarian cancer; can aid selection of patients who might benefit from secondary cytoreduction

Study: AGO DESKTOP OVAR III

- **Citation:** (Harter et al., 2021)
- **Highlight:** Secondary cytoreduction

- **Design:**
  - 407 patients with first recurrence of platinum-sensitive ovarian cancer and positive AGO score randomized to CT vs. secondary debulking followed by CT
  - CT at investigator's discretion
  - Positive AGO score
    - ECOG: 0
    - No residual tumor after primary surgery
    - No ascites (<500 cc, based on radiological estimate)
- **Results:**
  - Post-randomization CT in 90% platinum based in both groups
  - Macroscopic complete resection in 75.5%
  - Adjuvant BEV in 23%
  - Median follow-up: 69.8 months
  - Median OS: 53.7 vs. 46 months (surgery vs. CT) (HR: 0.75 [CI = 0.59–0.96]; p = 0.02)
    - Median OS: 61.9 vs. 27.7 months (complete resection vs. incomplete resection)
  - Median PFS overall: 18.4 vs. 14 months (HR 0.66 [CI = 0.54–0.82])
    - Median PFS in completely resected patients: 21.2 vs. 13.7 months (with residual tumor) and vs. 14 months (with CT only)
  - Median time to third line: 21 vs. 13.9 months
  - Quality of life through 1 yr did not differ
- **Conclusion:**
  - → Cytoreductive surgery followed by CT resulted in longer OS

Study: GOG 213

- **Citation:** (Coleman et al., 2019)
- **Highlight:** Secondary cytoreduction in recurrent platinum-sensitive ovarian cancer
- **Design:**
  - Bifactorial phase III trial with BEV objective and secondary cytoreduction objective; here, secondary cytoreduction objective reported
  - In December 2007 to June 2017, 485 patients with investigator-determined resectable platinum-sensitive ovarian cancer randomized to secondary cytoreduction followed by platinum-based CT vs. platinum-based CT alone
  - Stratified by platinum-free interval
- **Results:**
  - 215/240 (90%) randomized to secondary cytoreduction underwent the procedure
  - Complete resection achieved in 67%
  - Adjuvant BEV in 84%
  - Median follow-up: 48.1 months

- Median OS: 50.6 vs. 64.7 months (secondary cytoreduction vs. none) (HR for death 1.29 [CI = 0.97–1.72]; p = 0.08)
- Median PFS: 18.9 vs. 16.2 months (HR 0.82 [CI = 0.66–1.01])
- Patient-reported quality of life decreased significantly after surgery but did not differ after recovery
- **Conclusion:**
  - → Secondary cytoreduction can be safely performed but did not improve OS

Study: SOC-1

- **Citation:** (Shi et al., 2021)
- **Highlight:** Secondary cytoreduction in recurrent platinum-sensitive ovarian cancer
- **Design:**
  - 357 patients with platinum-sensitive recurrent ovarian cancer predicted to have resectable disease based on international model (iMODEL) and PET-CT randomized to CT vs. secondary debulking followed by CT
  - iMODEL score: stage, residual disease after primary surgery, platinum-free interval, ECOG status, Ca-125 at recurrence, and presence of ascites
  - Platinum-based doublet CT
- **Results:**
  - Median follow-up: 36.0 months
  - Median PFS: 17.4 vs. 11.9 months (surgery vs. no surgery)
  - At interim analysis, median OS: 58.1 vs. 53.9 months
- **Conclusion:**
  - → Secondary cytoreduction followed by CT associated with significantly longer PFS; OS will be assessed with mature data

2.1.9 Studies Addressing Treatment of Recurrent Ovarian Cancer, Platinum Resistant

2.1.9.1 Chemotherapy and Targeted Therapy

Study: GOG 170D

- **Citation:** (Burger et al., 2007)
- **Highlight:** Single-agent BEV
- **Design:**
  - Phase II trial: 62 patients with persistent or recurrent ovarian cancer with one or two prior regimens, measurable disease, and GOG performance status of at least two received BEV 15 mg/kg q 3 wks
- **Results:**
  - 66% received two prior regimens

- 58% platinum resistant
- Toxicities
  - Grade 3 HTN: 6/61
- ORR: 21% (2 CR; 11 PR)
- Median DOR: 10 months
- Median PFS: 4.7 months
- Median OS: 17 months
- **Conclusion:**
  - No significant association of platinum sensitivity, age, number of prior regimens, and performance status
  - → BEV well tolerated and active in second- and third-line treatments

Study: Cannistra trial

- **Citation:** (Cannistra et al., 2007)
- **Highlight:** Single-agent BEV
- **Design:**
  - Phase II trial: 44 patients with platinum-resistant ovarian cancer who progressed during or within 3 months of discontinuing topotecan or liposomal doxorubicin, and no more than three prior regimens received BEV 15 mg/kg q 3 wks
- **Results:**
  - Median of 5 C given
  - Grade 3–4 HTN: 9.1%
  - Proteinuria: 15.9%
  - Wound-healing complications: 2.3%
  - GI perforations: 11.4% (23.8% with three prior lines; 0% with two prior lines; $p < 0.01$)
  - Arterial thromboembolic events: 6.8%
  - Three deaths related to BEV
  - PR: 15.9%
  - Median PFS: 4.4 months
  - Median OS: 10.7 months
- **Conclusion:**
  - → BEV with single-agent activity in platinum-resistant ovarian cancer; higher than expected incidence of GI perforation noted in these heavily pretreated patients

Study: AURELIA trial

- **Citation:** (Pujade-Lauraine et al., 2014)
- **Highlight:** Single-agent CT ± BEV
- **Design:**
  - 361 patients with platinum-resistant ovarian cancer; after investigators selected CT regimen (i.e., PLD, weekly paclitaxel, or topotecan), patients

randomized to single-agent CT alone or with BEV (10 mg/kg q 2 wks or 15 mg/k q 3 wks)

- Crossover to single-agent BEV permitted after progression with CT alone
- Ineligible: patients with refractory disease, h/o bowel obstruction, or >2 prior regimens
- **Results:**
  - HTN ≥ grade 2 and proteinuria more common + BEV
  - GI perforations in 2.2% of BEV-treated patients
    - Median PFS: 6.7 vs. 3.4 months (p < 0.001) (+ BEV vs. – BEV)
  - ORR: 27.3% vs. 11.8% (p = 0.001)
  - Median OS: 16.6 vs. 13.3 months (p < 0.174)
- **Conclusion:**
  - → Adding BEV to CT improved PFS and ORR; trend in OS, no new safety signals

Study: AURELIA trial exploratory analysis

- **Citation:** (Poveda et al., 2015)
- **Highlight:** Weekly paclitaxel + BEV
- **Design:**
  - Exploratory subgroup analysis of the AURELIA trial data
- **Results:**
  - ORR Taxol group: 53.3% vs. 30.2% (+ vs. – BEV)
  - ORR topotecan group: 17% vs. 0%
  - ORR PLD group: 13.7% vs. 7.8%
  - Median OS: 22.4 vs. 13.8 vs. 13.7 months (paclitaxel + BEV vs. PLD + BEV vs. topotecan + BEV)
- **Conclusion:**
  - → Hypothesis generating on potential differences between the three regimens

Study: AURELIA trial exploratory analysis

- **Citation:** (Bamias et al., 2017)
- **Highlight:** Exploratory analysis given high crossover
- **Design:**
  - Exploratory analysis of patients who were randomized to CT alone
- **Results:**
  - Crossover: 72/182 received BEV after progression of disease on CT and 110 never received BEV
  - No significant differences in patient characteristics
  - Compared with patients never receiving BEV, risk of death reduced in patients receiving BEV upfront (HR = 0.68 [CI = 0.52–0.9]) or after progression of disease (HD = 0.6 [CI = 0.43–0.86])
  - Tolerability after progression of disease similar to upfront

- **Conclusion:**
  - → Post-progression of disease BEV application may have confounded OS results in AURELIA
  - Analysis of non-randomized subgroups; BEV either with CT or after progression of disease alone improved OS compared with no BEV
  - Combining BEV with CT at first appearance of platinum resistance maximizes likelihood of the effect of BEV

Study: FORWARD I

- **Citation:** (Moore et al., 2021b)
- **Highlight:** Mirvetuximab
- **Design:**
  - Mirvetuximab soravtansine (MIRV) = antibody-drug conjugate with folate receptor alpha (FRα)-binding antibody, a cleavable linker, and the maytansinoid DM4 (tubulin-targeting agent)
  - 366 patients with platinum-resistant ovarian cancer, one to three prior lines, and tumors positive for FRα randomized 2:1 to 6 mg/kg MIRV q 3 wks vs. CT (weekly paclitaxel 80 mg/m^2, doxil 40 mg/m^2, or weekly 4 mg/m^2 topotecan or 1.25 mg/m^2 topotecan on days 1–5 q 3 wks)
- **Results:**
  - Median PFS: 4.1 vs. 4.4 months (MIRV vs. CT)
    - In high FRα subgroup
      - Median PFS: 4.8 vs. 3.3 months
      - ORR: 24% vs. 10%
      - Ca-125 responses: 53% vs. 25%
      - Patient-reported outcomes (27% vs. 13%)
  - ≥ Grade 3 AEs: 25.1% vs. 44%
- **Conclusion:**
  - → MIRV did not result in improved PFS; secondary endpoints favored MIRV, particularly in patients with high FRα

Study: MIRASOL

- **Citation:** Ongoing (NCT04209855)
- **Highlight:** Mirvetuximab in FRα-high ovarian cancers
- **Design:**
  - Patients with platinum-resistant ovarian cancer with high FRα expression randomized to 6 mg/kg MIRV q 3 wks vs. CT (weekly paclitaxel 80 mg/m^2, doxil 40 mg/m^2, or weekly 4 mg/m^2 topotecan or 1.25 mg/m^2 topotecan on days 1–5 q 3 wks)

2.1.9.2 Immunotherapy

Study: Keynote-100

- **Citation:** (Matulonis et al., 2019)

- **Highlight:** Pembrolizumab in advanced recurrent ovarian cancer
- **Design:**
  - Two-cohort phase 2 trial: 285 (cohort A) and 91 (cohort B) patients with recurrent ovarian cancer received 200 mg pembrolizumab iv q 3 wks
    – Cohort A: One to three prior CT lines and platinum-/treatment-free interval between 3 and 12 months
    – Cohort B: Four to six prior CT lines and platinum-/treatment-free interval of ≥3 months
- **Results:**
  - 77% with high-grade serous histology
  - ORR: 7.4% for cohort A and 9.9% for cohort B
    – ORR in patients with CPS <1: 4.1%
    – ORR in patients with CPS ≥1: 5.7%
    – ORR in patients with CPS ≥10: 10%
  - Median DOR: 8.2 months for cohort A and not reached for cohort B
  - DCR: 47.2% for cohort A and 37.4% for cohort B
  - 19.7% with grade 3 and 4 AEs
  - Two deaths due to Stevens–Johnson syndrome and hypoaldosteronism
- **Conclusion:**
  - → Pembrolizumab with modest antitumor activity in recurrent ovarian cancer; ORR increased with PD-L1 expression

Study: TOPACIO/Keynote-162

- **Citation:** (Konstantinopoulos et al., 2019)
- **Highlight:** Niraparib and pembrolizumab
- **Design:**
  - In phase 1/2 trial, 60 patients with recurrent EOC irrespective of BRCA status, including platinum resistant (primary platinum refractory excluded, not secondary platinum refractory) received niraparib 200 mg qd po and pembrolizumab 200 mg iv q 3 wks
  - Somatic mutation testing for BRCA and homologous recombination deficiency (HRD) testing
- **Results:**
  - Median prior lines: Three
  - 63% had received BEV in prior treatment
  - 48% with platinum-resistant and 27% with platinum-refractory disease
  - Most common ≥ grade 3 AEs: Anemia (21%) and thrombocytopenia (9%)
  - Overall
    – ORR: 18%
    – DCR: 65%
    – Median DOR not reached
  - Subgroups
    – Platinum resistant: ORR 21% (6/29)
    – Platinum refractory: ORR 13% (2/16)
    – tBRCAmut: ORR 18% (2/11)

- tBRCAwt: ORR 19% (9/47)
- HRD positive: 14% (3/21)
- HRD negative: 19% (6/32)
- PD-L1 positive: 21% (7/33)
- PD-L1 negative: 10% (2/20)
- **Conclusion:**
  - → Niraparib plus pembrolizumab promising antitumor activity regardless of BRCA or biomarker status

Study: NRG-GY003

- **Citation:** (Zamarin et al., 2020)
- **Highlight:** Ipilimumab + nivolumab
- **Design:**
  - In randomized phase II trial, 100 patients with persistent or recurrent EOC and one to three prior lines randomized to nivolumab 3 mg/kg iv over 60 min q 2 wks × 4 doses followed by nivolumab maintenance 3 mg/kg iv over 60 min q 2 wks × up to 42 doses vs. nivolumab 3 mg/kg iv over 60 min plus ipilimumab 1 mg/kg iv over 90 min q 3 wks × 4 doses followed by nivolumab maintenance 3 mg/kg iv over 60 min q 2 wks × up to 42 doses
- **Results:**
  - 82% with high-grade serous histology
  - 62% with progression-free interval of <6 months
  - ORR: 12.2% (6/49) vs. 31.4% (16/51) (p = 0.034) (nivolumab vs. nivolumab + ipilimumab)
  - Median PFS: 2 vs. 3.9 months
  - Grade ≥3 AEs: 55% (27/49) vs. 67% (34/51); no treatment-related deaths
- **Conclusion:**
  - → Ipilimumab/nivolumab induction followed by nivolumab maintenance in patients with persistent or recurrent ovarian cancer superior to nivolumab alone, with albeit limited PFS

Study: LEAP-005 (NCT03797326), ongoing

- **Citation:** Abstract, presented at ESMO (2020), (Lwin et al., 2020)
- **Highlight:** Pembro/Lenvima
- **Design:**
  - In open-label multicohort study, patients with advanced pretreated solid tumors received lenvatinib 20 mg qd and pembrolizumab 200 mg q 3 wks
- **Results:**
  - 31 patients in ovarian cancer cohort
  - ORR: 32%
  - DCR: 74%
  - Grade ≥3 AEs: 68%

- Discontinued due to treatment-related AE: 13%
- **Conclusion:**
  - → Promising antitumor activity and manageable toxicity

Study: Zsiros trial

- **Citation:** (Zsiros et al., 2021)
- **Highlight:** Pembrolizumab, BEV, and oral metronomic cyclophosphamide
- **Design:**
  - In a phase II trial, 40 patients with recurrent ovarian cancer received 200 mg pembrolizumab iv q 3 wks and BEV 15 mg/kg iv q 3 wks plus 50 mg po cyclophosphamide qd
- **Results:**
  - 30 patients with platinum-resistant and 10 with platinum-sensitive disease
  - ORR: 47.5%
    - CR: 7.5%
    - PR: 40%
  - CBR: 95%
    - SD: 47.5%
  - Median PFS: 10 months
  - ≥Grade 3 AEs: Hypertension (15%) and lymphopenia (7.5%)
- **Conclusion:**
  - → The combination was well tolerated and showed CBR of 95% with durable response (>12 months) in 25% of patients

Study: IMagyn050/GOG 3015

- **Citation:** (Moore et al., 2021a)
- **Highlight:** Atezolizumab and BEV plus CT
- **Design:**
  - 1,301 patients with newly diagnosed stage III or IV ovarian cancer either s/p primary cytoreductive surgery with macroscopic residual disease or planned for NACT and IDS randomized to 1,200 mg atezolizumab q 3 wks plus carboplatin AUC 6, paclitaxel 175 mg/m², 15 mg/kg BEV vs. placebo plus carboplatin AUC 6, paclitaxel 175 mg/m², 15 mg/kg BEV, followed by atezolizumab vs. placebo plus BEV for 16 cycles
  - Atezolizumab = anti-PD-L1 antibody
- **Results:**
  - In intention-to-treat population
    - Median PFS: 19.5 vs. 18.4 months (HR 0.92 [CI = 0.79–1.07]; p = 0.28) (atezolizumab vs. placebo)
  - In PD-L1-positive population (≥1%)
    - Median PFS: 10.8 vs. 18.5 months (HR 0.8 [CI = 0.65–0.99]; p = 0.038)
  - ≥ Grade 3 AEs: Neutropenia (21% vs. 21%), hypertension (18% vs. 20%), and anemia (12% vs. 12%)

- **Conclusion:**
  - → Current evidence does not support use of immune checkpoint inhibitors in newly diagnosed ovarian cancer

Study: JAVELIN 100

- **Citation:** (Monk et al., 2021)
- **Highlight:** Avelumab plus CT
- **Design:**
  - 988 patients with stage III and IV ovarian cancer (following debulking surgery or candidates for NACT) randomized to six C of carboplatin AUC 5 or 6 and 175 mg/m² paclitaxel q 3 wks or 80 mg/m² q wk followed by avelumab 10 mg/kg iv q 2 wks (maintenance group) vs. CT plus avelumab 10 mg/kg iv q 3 wks followed by avelumab maintenance (combination group) vs. CT followed by observation (control group)
  - Avelumab = anti-PD-L1 antibody
- **Results:**
  - At interim analysis, prespecified futility boundaries were crossed and trial stopped
  - Median PFS: NE (not estimable) vs. 16.8 vs. 18.1 months (control vs. maintenance vs. combination)
  - Stratified HR: 1.43 for maintenance vs. control and 1.14 for combination vs. control
- **Conclusion:**
  - Results do not support use of avelumab in frontline setting for patients with advanced ovarian cancer

2.2 LOW-GRADE SEROUS OVARIAN CANCER

Study: Gershenson study

- **Citation:** (Gershenson et al., 2017)
- **Highlight:** Hormonal maintenance
- **Design:**
  - Retrospective study on 203 patients with stage II–IV low-grade serous ovarian cancer s/p primary surgery followed by platinum-based CT
  - Hormonal maintenance therapy (HMT): 54.3% letrozole, 2.9% anastrozole, 28.6% tamoxifen, and 7.1% leuprolide acetate (the latter plus letrozole, tamoxifen, or depot medroxyprogesterone acetate)
- **Results:**
  - 133 patients underwent observation; 70 received HMT
  - Median PFS: 26.4 vs. 64.9 months (p < 0.001) (observation vs. HMT)
  - Median OS: 102.7 vs. 115.7 months

- In disease-free: Median PFS: 30 vs. 81.1 months
- With persistent disease: Median PFS: 15.2 vs. 38.1 months
- With HMT lower risk of disease progression: HR 0.44 [CI = 0.31–0.64]; p < 0.001
- **Conclusion:**
  - → In low-grade serous ovarian cancer significantly longer PFS with HMT

Study: MSKCC series

- **Citation:** (Grisham et al., 2014)
- **Highlight:** CT plus BEV in recurrent disease
- **Design:**
  - Retrospective study on 15 patients with recurrent low-grade serous ovarian cancer; two patients received single-agent BEV; the remainder BEV plus CT (paclitaxel, topotecan, oral cyclophosphamide, gemcitabine, or gemcitabine and carboplatin)
- **Results:**
  - ORR: 55%
  - CR: None
  - PR in six patients
- **Conclusion:**
  - → BEV plus CT is active treatment in recurrent low-grade serous ovarian cancer

Study: GOG 281

- **Citation:** (Gershenson et al., 2022)
- **Highlight:** Trametinib
- **Background:** Low-grade serous ovarian cancer characterized by MAPK pathway aberrations and reduced sensitivity to CT
- **Design:**
  - 260 patients with recurrent low-grade serous carcinoma with measurable disease and at least one platinum-based regimen randomized to 2 mg trametinib qd vs. standard of care (paclitaxel 80 mg/m^2 on days 1, 8, and 15 of 28 d cycle; doxil 40–50 mg/m^2 q 28 d; topotecan 4 mg/m^2 on days 1, 8, and 15 of 28 d cycle; oral 2.5 mg letrozole qd; oral tamoxifen 20 mg q 12 hrs)
  - Stratified by geographical region, number of previous regimens, performance status, and standard-of-care regimen
- **Results:**
  - Median follow-up: 31.3 months
  - ORR: 26% vs. 6% (trametinib vs. standard of care)
  - Median DOR: 13.6 vs. 5.9 months
  - Median PFS: 13.0 vs. 7.2 months (HR 0.48 [CI = 0.36–0.64]; p < 0.0001)

- Post hoc analysis of median PFS
  - 15.0 vs. 10.6 months (trametinib vs. letrozole)
  - 11.8 vs. 10.0 months (trametinib vs. doxil)
  - 9.5 vs. 5.0 months (trametinib vs. weekly Taxol)
  - 9.8 vs. 3.1 months (trametinib vs. topotecan)
  - 19.1 vs. 3.7 months (trametinib vs. tamoxifen)
- Most frequent grade 3 AEs
  - In the trametinib group: Skin rash (13%), anemia (13%), hypertension (12%), and diarrhea (10%)
- **Conclusion:**
  - → Trametinib new standard of care for recurrent low-grade serous ovarian carcinoma

2.3 MUCINOUS EPITHELIAL OVARIAN CANCER

Study: GOG 241

- **Citation:** (Gore et al., 2019)
- **Background:**
  - Advanced mucinous epithelial ovarian cancer (mEOC) responds only poorly to standard CT; only <8% patients in ovarian cancer trials (difficult to examine this subgroup); here, first-ever randomized trial for this rare subgroup
- **Design:**
  - 50 patients with advanced or recurrent mEOC, chemo-naïve randomized to four CT regimens; stopped early (2013) because of slow accrual
  - Intended: 332 patients required to detect 5-month increase in PFS
  - Regimens
    - A: Carboplatin AUC 5/6 plus paclitaxel 175 mg/m^2 q 3 wks × 6 C
    - B: Oxaliplatin 130 mg/m^2 plus capecitabine 850 mg/m^2 BID days 1–14
    - C: Carboplatin AUC 5/6 plus paclitaxel 175 mg/m^2 plus BEV 15 mg/kg q 3 wks × 6 C
    - D: Oxaliplatin 130 mg/m^2 plus capecitabine 850 mg/m^2 BID days 1–14 plus BEV 15 mg/kg
    - BEV given concurrently, then alone 3-weekly for 12 more cycles
- **Results:**
  - Median follow-up: 59 months
  - OS HR: 0.78 (p = 0.48) for B vs. A, and 1.04 (p = 0.92) for BEV vs. no BEV
  - PFS HR: 0.84 for B vs. A, and 0.8 for BEV vs. no BEV
  - Central pathology review: Only 45% (18/40) confirmed primary mEOC

- – Among these: OS HR: 0.36 (p = 0.14) for B vs. A, and PFS HR 0.62 (p = 0.4)
  - Grade 3–4 toxicities (most common: neutropenia and HTN for BEV) seen in 61%, 61%, 54%, and 85% in A–D
- **Conclusion:**
  - → Logistical challenges; rare cancer trials should include centralized pathology review; no therapeutic conclusion can be made

Study: Cho retrospective study

- **Citation:** (Cho et al., 2006)
- **Highlight:** Value of complete staging in mEOC
- **Design:**
  - Retrospective study to evaluate the impact on prognosis of complete surgical staging with stage I mucinous ovarian tumors
  - Of 264 patients, 23.5% had complete and 76.5% incomplete initial surgical staging
- **Results:**
  - No patient with clinically apparent stage I borderline tumor upstaged
  - 5/85 patients with invasive mucinous cancer upstaged due to positive peritoneal cytology
  - No patient upstaged due to occult LN metastasis
  - No recurrence in completely staged; two (1.4%) in incompletely staged patients with borderline tumors
  - Three (11.5%) recurrences in completely staged and four (6.8%) incompletely staged patients with invasive cancers (difference not significant)
  - Also, no difference in PFS and OS
- **Conclusion:**
  - → Complete surgical staging could be omitted in patients with clinical stage I mEOCs

Study: Schmeler retrospective study

- **Citation:** (Schmeler et al., 2010)
- **Highlight:** Prevalence of positive LNs in early-stage mEOC
- **Design:**
  - Retrospective study to estimate prevalence of LN metastases in primary mEOC
- **Results:**
  - 107 patients with primary mEOC identified
  - 93/107 (87%) at time of surgery grossly confined to the ovary and 14/107 with extraovarian disease
  - 51/93 (55%) underwent lymphadenectomy
    - – None with PA or PLN metastasis
    - – No differences in PFS and OS between patients who underwent lymphadenectomy and those who did not

- **Conclusion:**
  - → No cases of isolated LN metastasis with primary mEOC grossly confined to the ovary, suggesting that routine lymphadenectomy may be omitted in these patients

2.4 SMALL-CELL CARCINOMA OF THE OVARY

Study: Senekjian case report

- **Citation:** (Senekjian et al., 1989)
- **Highlight:** VPCBAE in small-cell carcinoma of the ovary (SCCO)
- **Design:**
  - Case report of two patients with stage IA, one stage IIC and two stage IIIA small-cell cancer of the ovary received adjuvant 6 mg/m^2 vinblastine and 90 mg/m^2 cisplatin at hour zero, 1 g/m^2 cyclophosphamide and 15 U/m^2 bleomycin at 24 hrs, and 60 mg/m^2 doxorubicin and 200 mg/m^2 etoposide at 36 hrs every 3–4 wks
- **Results:**
  - The two patients who had measurable disease showed objective responses
  - 4/5 patients died 11–18 months after initial laparotomy
  - 1/5 patients alive and disease-free after 29 months
- **Conclusion:**
  - → VPCBAE appears effective in select cases of SCCO. Further studies seem to be indicated

2.5 OVARIAN GERM CELL TUMORS

Study: GOG 45

- **Citation:** (Williams et al., 1989)
- **Highlight:** Cisplatin/vinblastine/bleomycin (PVB)
- **Design:**
  - Non-randomized prospective trial: 97 patients with advanced ovarian germ cell tumors received 3–4 C of PVB
  - After CT, suitable patients underwent restaging exlap
  - Maintenance vinblastine originally given but discontinued in 1981
  - Patients with persistent or recurrent disease treated with vincristine, dactinomycin, and cyclophosphamide (VAC) or etoposide plus cisplatin (EP)

- **Results:**
  - Eight dysgerminomas; 89 other cell types
  - 15/35 with tumors other than dysgerminoma who had measurable disease with CR
  - 40/56 second look exlap: No tumor or mature teratoma
  - 2-yr PFS: 51%
  - 2-yr OS: 71%
  - Eight patients with durable remissions with second- and third-line therapies
  - 7/8 with dysgerminomas disease-free
- **Conclusion:**
  - → Cisplatin-based CT effective for ovarian germ cell tumors and superior to previous regimens and will cure a substantial number

Study: GOG 78

- **Citation:** (Williams et al., 1994)
- **Highlight:** Bleomycin/etoposide/cisplatin (BEP)
- **Design:**
  - To determine the effectiveness of postoperative adjuvant CT
  - Non-randomized prospective trial: 93 patients with surgically staged and completely resected ovarian germ cell tumors received BEP × 3 C, then second-look exlap
- **Results:**
  - Acute toxicity: Moderate
  - One patient developed AML 22 months after diagnosis; one patient a malignant lymphoma 69 months post-treatment
  - 89/93 remained free of germ cell cancer
  - 2/93 with small foci of immature teratoma (both remained clinically free of recurrence; one received alternate CT; one did not)
  - 67 patients had been monitored over 2 yrs at the time of publication
- **Conclusion:**
  - → 3 C of BEP will nearly always prevent recurrence in staged and completely resected ovarian germ cell tumors

2.6 OVARIAN SEX CORD-STROMAL TUMORS

Study: PARAGON

- **Citation:** (Banerjee et al., 2021)
- **Highlight:** Anastrozole in metastatic granulosa cell tumor

- **Background:**
  - Granulosa cell tumors frequently strongly express ER and/or PR and are commonly treated with anti-estrogens
  - Pooled response rates based on case reports and retrospective series: 70%; aromatase inhibitors reported especially effective
- **Design:**
  - Phase II: 41 postmenopausal patients with ER/PR + metastatic granulosa cell tumor and measurable disease and/or elevated inhibin received anastrozole 1 mg qd po until progression or toxicity
- **Results:**
  - 3-month CBR: 78.9%
    - PR: 2.6%
    - SD: 76.3%
    - Delayed response after 3 months with PR: Four patients
  - PD: 20%
  - Median PFS: 8.6 months
  - 6-month PFS: 59%
  - Grade 3 AE: One patient with arthralgia
- **Conclusion:**
  - → Although high CBR, ORR much lower than historical pooled results

Study: GOG 264

- **Citation:** Ongoing (NCT01042522)
- **Highlight:** Carbo/Taxol vs. BEP in SCTs
- **Design:**
  - Phase II trial: Patients with newly diagnosed stage IIA–IV ovarian stromal tumor within 8 wks after surgery with measurable or no measurable disease or biopsy-proven recurrence and chemo-naïve randomized to carboplatin over 1 hr and paclitaxel over 3 hrs q 3 wks × 6 C vs. bleomycin sulfate over 1 hr on day 1 and etoposide over 1 hr on day 1 and cisplatin iv over 30 min on days 1–5 q 3 wks × 4 C
  - Opened in 2010, accrual goal 128 patients; in 2016, 35 enrolled

REFERENCES

Aghajanian, C., Blank, S.V., Goff, B.A., Judson, P.L., Teneriello, M.G., Husain, A., Sovak, M.A., Yi, J., and Nycum, L.R. (2012). OCEANS: a randomized, double-blind, placebo-controlled phase III trial of chemotherapy with or without bevacizumab in patients with platinum-sensitive recurrent epithelial ovarian, primary peritoneal, or fallopian tube cancer. J Clin Oncol *30*, 2039–2045. 10.1200/JCO.2012.42.0505.

Aghajanian, C., Goff, B., Nycum, L.R., Wang, Y.V., Husain, A., and Blank, S.V. (2015). Final overall survival and safety analysis of OCEANS, a phase 3 trial of chemotherapy with or without bevacizumab in patients with platinum-sensitive recurrent ovarian cancer. Gynecol Oncol *139*, 10–16. 10.1016/j.ygyno.2015.08.004.

Alberts, D.S., Liu, P.Y., Hannigan, E.V., O'Toole, R., Williams, S.D., Young, J.A., Franklin, E.W., Clarke-Pearson, D.L., Malviya, V.K., and DuBeshter, B. (1996). Intraperitoneal cisplatin plus intravenous cyclophosphamide versus intravenous cisplatin plus intravenous cyclophosphamide for stage III ovarian cancer. N Engl J Med *335*, 1950–1955. 10.1056/NEJM199612263352603.

Armstrong, D.K., Bundy, B., Wenzel, L., Huang, H.Q., Baergen, R., Lele, S., Copeland, L.J., Walker, J.L., Burger, R.A., and Gynecologic Oncology Group. (2006). Intraperitoneal cisplatin and paclitaxel in ovarian cancer. N Engl J Med *354*, 34–43. 10.1056/NEJMoa052985.

Bamias, A., Gibbs, E., Khoon Lee, C., Davies, L., Dimopoulos, M., Zagouri, F., Veillard, A.S., Kosse, J., Santaballa, A., Mirza, M.R., et al. (2017). Bevacizumab with or after chemotherapy for platinum-resistant recurrent ovarian cancer: exploratory analyses of the AURELIA trial. Ann Oncol *28*, 1842–1848. 10.1093/annonc/mdx228.

Banerjee, S.N., Tang, M., O'Connell, R.L., Sjoquist, K., Clamp, A.R., Millan, D., Nottley, S., Lord, R., Mullassery, V.M., Hall, M., et al. (2021). A phase 2 study of anastrozole in patients with oestrogen receptor and/progesterone receptor positive recurrent/metastatic granulosa cell tumours/sex-cord stromal tumours of the ovary: the PARAGON/ANZGOG 0903 trial. Gynecol Oncol *163*, 72–78. 10.1016/j.ygyno.2021.07.024.

Bell, J., Brady, M.F., Young, R.C., Lage, J., Walker, J.L., Look, K.Y., Rose, G.S., Spirtos, N.M., and Gynecologic Oncology Group. (2006). Randomized phase III trial of three versus six cycles of adjuvant carboplatin and paclitaxel in early stage epithelial ovarian carcinoma: a Gynecologic Oncology Group study. Gynecol Oncol *102*, 432–439. 10.1016/j.ygyno.2006.06.013.

Bookman, M.A., Brady, M.F., McGuire, W.P., Harper, P.G., Alberts, D.S., Friedlander, M., Colombo, N., Fowler, J.M., Argenta, P.A., De Geest, K., et al. (2009). Evaluation of new platinum-based treatment regimens in advanced-stage ovarian cancer: a phase III trial of the gynecologic cancer intergroup. J Clin Oncol *27*, 1419–1425. 10.1200/JCO.2008.19.1684.

Burger, R.A., Brady, M.F., Bookman, M.A., Fleming, G.F., Monk, B.J., Huang, H., Mannel, R.S., Homesley, H.D., Fowler, J., Greer, B.E., et al. (2011). Incorporation of bevacizumab in the primary treatment of ovarian cancer. N Engl J Med *365*, 2473–2483. 10.1056/NEJMoa1104390.

Burger, R.A., Sill, M.W., Monk, B.J., Greer, B.E., and Sorosky, J.I. (2007). Phase II trial of bevacizumab in persistent or recurrent epithelial ovarian cancer or primary peritoneal cancer: a Gynecologic Oncology Group study. J Clin Oncol *25*, 5165–5171. 10.1200/JCO.2007.11.5345.

Cannistra, S.A., Matulonis, U.A., Penson, R.T., Hambleton, J., Dupont, J., Mackey, H., Douglas, J., Burger, R.A., Armstrong, D., Wenham, R., and McGuire, W. (2007). Phase II study of bevacizumab in patients with platinum-resistant ovarian cancer or peritoneal serous cancer. J Clin Oncol *25*, 5180–5186. 10.1200/JCO.2007.12.0782.

Chan, J.K., Brady, M.F., Penson, R.T., Huang, H., Birrer, M.J., Walker, J.L., DiSilvestro, P.A., Rubin, S.C., Martin, L.P., Davidson, S.A., et al. (2016). Weekly vs. every-3-week paclitaxel and carboplatin for ovarian cancer. N Engl J Med *374*, 738–748. 10.1056/NEJMoa1505067.

Cho, Y.H., Kim, D.Y., Kim, J.H., Kim, Y.M., Kim, K.R., Kim, Y.T., and Nam, J.H. (2006). Is complete surgical staging necessary in patients with stage I mucinous epithelial ovarian tumors? Gynecol Oncol *103*, 878–882. 10.1016/j.ygyno.2006.05.022.

Clamp, A.R., James, E.C., McNeish, I.A., Dean, A., Kim, J.W., O'Donnell, D.M., Hook, J., Coyle, C., Blagden, S., Brenton, J.D., et al. (2019). Weekly dose-dense chemotherapy in first-line epithelial ovarian, fallopian tube, or primary peritoneal carcinoma treatment (ICON8):

primary progression free survival analysis results from a GCIG phase 3 randomised controlled trial. Lancet *394*, 2084–2095. 10.1016/S0140–6736(19)32259-7.

Coleman, R.L., Brady, M.F., Herzog, T.J., Sabbatini, P., Armstrong, D.K., Walker, J.L., Kim, B.G., Fujiwara, K., Tewari, K.S., O'Malley, D.M., et al. (2017a). Bevacizumab and paclitaxel-carboplatin chemotherapy and secondary cytoreduction in recurrent, platinum-sensitive ovarian cancer (NRG Oncology/Gynecologic Oncology Group study GOG-0213): a multicentre, open-label, randomised, phase 3 trial. Lancet Oncol *18*, 779–791. 10.1016/S1470–2045(17)30279-6.

Coleman, R.L., Oza, A.M., Lorusso, D., Aghajanian, C., Oaknin, A., Dean, A., Colombo, N., Weberpals, J.I., Clamp, A., Scambia, G., et al. (2017b). Rucaparib maintenance treatment for recurrent ovarian carcinoma after response to platinum therapy (ARIEL3): a randomised, double-blind, placebo-controlled, phase 3 trial. Lancet *390*, 1949–1961. 10.1016/S0140–6736(17)32440-6.

Coleman, R.L., Spirtos, N.M., Enserro, D., Herzog, T.J., Sabbatini, P., Armstrong, D.K., Kim, J.W., Park, S.Y., Kim, B.G., Nam, J.H., et al. (2019). Secondary surgical cytoreduction for recurrent ovarian cancer. N Engl J Med *381*, 1929–1939. 10.1056/NEJMoa1902626.

Colombo, N., Guthrie, D., Chiari, S., Parmar, M., Qian, W., Swart, A.M., Torri, V., Williams, C., Lissoni, A., Bonazzi, C., and International Collaborative Ovarian Neoplasm, c. (2003). International Collaborative Ovarian Neoplasm trial 1: a randomized trial of adjuvant chemotherapy in women with early-stage ovarian cancer. J Natl Cancer Inst *95*, 125–132.

Del Campo, J.M., Matulonis, U.A., Malander, S., Provencher, D., Mahner, S., Follana, P., Waters, J., Berek, J.S., Woie, K., Oza, A.M., et al. (2019). Niraparib maintenance therapy in patients with recurrent ovarian cancer after a partial response to the last platinum-based chemotherapy in the ENGOT-OV16/NOVA trial. J Clin Oncol *37*, 2968–2973. 10.1200/JCO.18.02238.

DiSilvestro, P., Colombo, N., Scambia, G., Kim, B.G., Oaknin, A., Friedlander, M., Lisyanskaya, A., Floquet, A., Leary, A., Sonke, G.S., et al. (2020). Efficacy of maintenance olaparib for patients with newly diagnosed advanced ovarian cancer with a BRCA mutation: subgroup analysis findings from the SOLO1 trial. J Clin Oncol *38*, 3528–3537. 10.1200/JCO.20.00799.

Domchek, S.M., Aghajanian, C., Shapira-Frommer, R., Schmutzler, R.K., Audeh, M.W., Friedlander, M., Balmana, J., Mitchell, G., Fried, G., Stemmer, S.M., et al. (2016). Efficacy and safety of olaparib monotherapy in germline BRCA1/2 mutation carriers with advanced ovarian cancer and three or more lines of prior therapy. Gynecol Oncol *140*, 199–203. 10.1016/j.ygyno.2015.12.020.

du Bois, A., Reuss, A., Harter, P., Pujade-Lauraine, E., Ray-Coquard, I., Pfisterer, J., Arbeitsgemeinschaft Gynaekologische Onkologie Studiengruppe, O., and Groupe d'Investigateurs Nationaux pour l'Etude des Cancers, O. (2010). Potential role of lymphadenectomy in advanced ovarian cancer: a combined exploratory analysis of three prospectively randomized phase III multicenter trials. J Clin Oncol *28*, 1733–1739. 10.1200/JCO.2009.25.3617.

Fagotti, A., Ferrandina, G., Fanfani, F., Garganese, G., Vizzielli, G., Carone, V., Salerno, M.G., and Scambia, G. (2008). Prospective validation of a laparoscopic predictive model for optimal cytoreduction in advanced ovarian carcinoma. Am J Obstet Gynecol *199*, 642 e641–646. 10.1016/j.ajog.2008.06.052.

Fagotti, A., Ferrandina, G., Vizzielli, G., Fanfani, F., Gallotta, V., Chiantera, V., Costantini, B., Margariti, P.A., Gueli Alletti, S., Cosentino, F., et al. (2016). Phase III randomised clinical trial comparing primary surgery versus neoadjuvant chemotherapy in advanced epithelial ovarian cancer with high tumour load (SCORPION trial): final analysis of peri-operative outcome. Eur J Cancer *59*, 22–33. 10.1016/j.ejca.2016.01.017.

Fagotti, A., Ferrandina, M.G., Vizzielli, G., Pasciuto, T., Fanfani, F., Gallotta, V., Margariti, P.A., Chiantera, V., Costantini, B., Gueli Alletti, S., et al. (2020). Randomized trial of primary debulking surgery versus neoadjuvant chemotherapy for advanced epithelial ovarian cancer (SCORPION-NCT01461850). Int J Gynecol Cancer 30, 1657–1664. 10.1136/ijgc-2020-001640.

Friedlander, M., Moore, K.N., Colombo, N., Scambia, G., Kim, B.G., Oaknin, A., Lisyanskaya, A., Sonke, G.S., Gourley, C., Banerjee, S., et al. (2021). Patient-centred outcomes and effect of disease progression on health status in patients with newly diagnosed advanced ovarian cancer and a BRCA mutation receiving maintenance olaparib or placebo (SOLO1): a randomised, phase 3 trial. Lancet Oncol 22, 632–642. 10.1016/S1470-2045(21)00098-X.

Gershenson, D.M., Bodurka, D.C., Coleman, R.L., Lu, K.H., Malpica, A., and Sun, C.C. (2017). Hormonal maintenance therapy for women with low-grade serous cancer of the ovary or peritoneum. J Clin Oncol 35, 1103–1111. 10.1200/JCO.2016.71.0632.

Gershenson, D.M., Miller, A., Brady, W.E., Paul, J., Carty, K., Rodgers, W., Millan, D., Coleman, R.L., Moore, K.N., Banerjee, S., et al. (2022). Trametinib versus standard of care in patients with recurrent low-grade serous ovarian cancer (GOG 281/LOGS): an international, randomised, open-label, multicentre, phase 2/3 trial. Lancet 399, 541–553. 10.1016/S0140-6736(21)02175-9.

Gonzalez-Martin, A., Pothuri, B., Vergote, I., DePont Christensen, R., Graybill, W., Mirza, M.R., McCormick, C., Lorusso, D., Hoskins, P., Freyer, G., et al. (2019). Niraparib in patients with newly diagnosed advanced ovarian cancer. N Engl J Med 381, 2391–2402. 10.1056/NEJMoa1910962.

Gordon, A.N., Fleagle, J.T., Guthrie, D., Parkin, D.E., Gore, M.E., and Lacave, A.J. (2001). Recurrent epithelial ovarian carcinoma: a randomized phase III study of pegylated liposomal doxorubicin versus topotecan. J Clin Oncol 19, 3312–3322. 10.1200/JCO.2001.19.14.3312.

Gore, M., Hackshaw, A., Brady, W.E., Penson, R.T., Zaino, R., McCluggage, W.G., Ganesan, R., Wilkinson, N., Perren, T., Montes, A., et al. (2019). An international, phase III randomized trial in patients with mucinous epithelial ovarian cancer (mEOC/GOG 0241) with long-term follow-up: and experience of conducting a clinical trial in a rare gynecological tumor. Gynecol Oncol 153, 541–548. 10.1016/j.ygyno.2019.03.256.

Grisham R.N., Iyer G., Sala E., Zhou Q., Iasonos A., DeLair D., Hyman D.M., and Aghajanian C. (2014). Bevacizumab shows activity in patients with low-grade serous ovarian and primary peritoneal cancer. Int J Gynecol Cancer 24(6), 1010–1014. PMID: 24978709.

Harter, P., du Bois, A., Hahmann, M., Hasenburg, A., Burges, A., Loibl, S., Gropp, M., Huober, J., Fink, D., Schroder, W., et al. (2006). Surgery in recurrent ovarian cancer: the arbeitsgemeinschaft gynaekologische onkologie (AGO) DESKTOP OVAR trial. Ann Surg Oncol 13, 1702–1710. 10.1245/s10434-006-9058-0.

Harter, P., Sehouli, J., Lorusso, D., Reuss, A., Vergote, I., Marth, C., Kim, J.W., Raspagliesi, F., Lampe, B., Aletti, G., et al. (2019). A randomized trial of lymphadenectomy in patients with advanced ovarian neoplasms. N Engl J Med 380, 822–832. 10.1056/NEJMoa1808424.

Harter, P., Sehouli, J., Reuss, A., Hasenburg, A., Scambia, G., Cibula, D., Mahner, S., Vergote, I., Reinthaller, A., Burges, A., et al. (2011). Prospective validation study of a predictive score for operability of recurrent ovarian cancer: the multicenter intergroup study DESKTOP II. A project of the AGO kommission OVAR, AGO study group, NOGGO, AGO-Austria, and MITO. Int J Gynecol Cancer 21, 289–295. 10.1097/IGC.0b013e31820aaafd.

Harter, P., Sehouli, J., Vergote, I., Ferron, G., Reuss, A., Meier, W., Greggi, S., Mosgard, B.J., Selle, F., Guyon, F., et al. (2021). Randomized trial of cytoreductive surgery for relapsed ovarian cancer. N Engl J Med 385, 2123–2131. 10.1056/NEJMoa2103294.

ICON2. (1998). Randomised trial of single-agent carboplatin against three-drug combination of CAP (cyclophosphamide, doxorubicin, and cisplatin) in women with ovarian cancer. ICON Collaborators. Int Collaborat Ovar Neoplasm Study. Lancet *352*, 1571–1576.

International Collaborative Ovarian Neoplasm, G. (2002). Paclitaxel plus carboplatin versus standard chemotherapy with either single-agent carboplatin or cyclophosphamide, doxorubicin, and cisplatin in women with ovarian cancer: the ICON3 randomised trial. Lancet *360*, 505–515. 10.1016/S0140–6736(02)09738-6.

Katsumata, N., Yasuda, M., Isonishi, S., Takahashi, F., Michimae, H., Kimura, E., Aoki, D., Jobo, T., Kodama, S., Terauchi, F., et al. (2013). Long-term results of dose-dense paclitaxel and carboplatin versus conventional paclitaxel and carboplatin for treatment of advanced epithelial ovarian, fallopian tube, or primary peritoneal cancer (JGOG 3016): a randomised, controlled, open-label trial. Lancet Oncol *14*, 1020–1026. 10.1016/S1470–2045(13)70363-2.

Katsumata, N., Yasuda, M., Takahashi, F., Isonishi, S., Jobo, T., Aoki, D., Tsuda, H., Sugiyama, T., Kodama, S., Kimura, E., et al. (2009). Dose-dense paclitaxel once a week in combination with carboplatin every 3 weeks for advanced ovarian cancer: a phase 3, open-label, randomised controlled trial. Lancet *374*, 1331–1338. 10.1016/S0140–6736(09)61157-0.

Kehoe, S., Hook, J., Nankivell, M., Jayson, G.C., Kitchener, H., Lopes, T., Luesley, D., Perren, T., Bannoo, S., Mascarenhas, M., et al. (2015). Primary chemotherapy versus primary surgery for newly diagnosed advanced ovarian cancer (CHORUS): an open-label, randomised, controlled, non-inferiority trial. Lancet *386*, 249–257. 10.1016/S0140–6736(14)62223-6.

Konstantinopoulos, P.A., Waggoner, S., Vidal, G.A., Mita, M., Moroney, J.W., Holloway, R., Van Le, L., Sachdev, J.C., Chapman-Davis, E., Colon-Otero, G., et al. (2019). Single-arm phases 1 and 2 trial of niraparib in combination with pembrolizumab in patients with recurrent platinum-resistant ovarian carcinoma. JAMA Oncol *5*(8), 1141–1149. 10.1001/jamaoncol.2019.1048.

Kristeleit, R., Lisyanskaya, A., Fedenko, A., Dvorkin, M., de Melo, A.C., Shparyk, Y., Rakhmatullina, I., Bondarenko, I., Colombo, N., Svintsitskiy, V., et al. (2022). Rucaparib versus standard-of-care chemotherapy in patients with relapsed ovarian cancer and a deleterious BRCA1 or BRCA2 mutation (ARIEL4): an international, open-label, randomised, phase 3 trial. Lancet Oncol *23*, 465–478. 10.1016/S1470–2045(22)00122-X.

Ledermann, J., Harter, P., Gourley, C., Friedlander, M., Vergote, I., Rustin, G., Scott, C.L., Meier, W., Shapira-Frommer, R., Safra, T., et al. (2012). Olaparib maintenance therapy in platinum-sensitive relapsed ovarian cancer. N Engl J Med *366*, 1382–1392. 10.1056/NEJMoa1105535.

Ledermann, J., Harter, P., Gourley, C., Friedlander, M., Vergote, I., Rustin, G., Scott, C.L., Meier, W., Shapira-Frommer, R., Safra, T., et al. (2014). Olaparib maintenance therapy in patients with platinum-sensitive relapsed serous ovarian cancer: a preplanned retrospective analysis of outcomes by BRCA status in a randomised phase 2 trial. Lancet Oncol *15*, 852–861. 10.1016/S1470–2045(14)70228-1.

Ledermann, J.A., Harter, P., Gourley, C., Friedlander, M., Vergote, I., Rustin, G., Scott, C., Meier, W., Shapira-Frommer, R., Safra, T., et al. (2016). Overall survival in patients with platinum-sensitive recurrent serous ovarian cancer receiving olaparib maintenance monotherapy: an updated analysis from a randomised, placebo-controlled, double-blind, phase 2 trial. Lancet Oncol *17*, 1579–1589. 10.1016/S1470-2045(16)30376-X.

Lwin, Z., Gomez-Rocan, C., Saada-Bouzid, E., Yanez, E., Longo Munoz, F., Im, S., Castanon, E., Senellart, H., Graham, D., Voss, M., Doherty, M., Lopez, J., Ghori, R., Kubiak, P., Jin,. F., Norwood, K., and Chung, H.C. (2020). LEAP-005: phase II study of lenvatinib (len) plus pembrolizumab (pembro) in patients (pts) with previously treated advanced solid tumours. In suppl_4. (Annals of Oncology), S1142–S1215.

Markman, M., Bundy, B.N., Alberts, D.S., Fowler, J.M., Clark-Pearson, D.L., Carson, L.F., Wadler, S., and Sickel, J. (2001). Phase III trial of standard-dose intravenous cisplatin plus paclitaxel versus moderately high-dose carboplatin followed by intravenous paclitaxel and intraperitoneal cisplatin in small-volume stage III ovarian carcinoma: an intergroup study of the Gynecologic Oncology Group, Southwestern Oncology Group, and Eastern Cooperative Oncology Group. J Clin Oncol 19, 1001–1007. 10.1200/JCO.2001.19.4.1001.

Markman, M., Liu, P.Y., Wilczynski, S., Monk, B., Copeland, L.J., Alvarez, R.D., Jiang, C., Alberts, D., Southwest Oncology Group, and Gynecologic Oncology Group. (2003). Phase III randomized trial of 12 versus 3 months of maintenance paclitaxel in patients with advanced ovarian cancer after complete response to platinum and paclitaxel-based chemotherapy: a Southwest Oncology Group and Gynecologic Oncology Group trial. J Clin Oncol 21, 2460–2465. 10.1200/JCO.2003.07.013.

Matulonis, U.A., Shapira-Frommer, R., Santin, A.D., Lisyanskaya, A.S., Pignata, S., Vergote, I., Raspagliesi, F., Sonke, G.S., Birrer, M., Provencher, D.M., et al. (2019). Antitumor activity and safety of pembrolizumab in patients with advanced recurrent ovarian cancer: results from the phase II KEYNOTE-100 study. Ann Oncol 30, 1080–1087. 10.1093/annonc/mdz135.

McGuire, W.P., Hoskins, W.J., Brady, M.F., Kucera, P.R., Partridge, E.E., Look, K.Y., Clarke-Pearson, D.L., and Davidson, M. (1996). Cyclophosphamide and cisplatin compared with paclitaxel and cisplatin in patients with stage III and stage IV ovarian cancer. N Engl J Med 334, 1–6. 10.1056/NEJM199601043340101.

Mirza, M.R., Avall Lundqvist, E., Birrer, M.J., dePont Christensen, R., Nyvang, G.B., Malander, S., Anttila, M., Werner, T.L., Lund, B., Lindahl, G., et al. (2019). Niraparib plus bevacizumab versus niraparib alone for platinum-sensitive recurrent ovarian cancer (NSGO-AVANOVA2/ENGOT-ov24): a randomised, phase 2, superiority trial. Lancet Oncol 20, 1409–1419. 10.1016/S1470-2045(19)30515-7.

Mirza, M.R., Monk, B.J., Herrstedt, J., Oza, A.M., Mahner, S., Redondo, A., Fabbro, M., Ledermann, J.A., Lorusso, D., Vergote, I., et al. (2016). Niraparib maintenance therapy in platinum-sensitive, recurrent ovarian cancer. N Engl J Med 375, 2154–2164. 10.1056/NEJMoa1611310.

Monk, B.J., Colombo, N., Oza, A.M., Fujiwara, K., Birrer, M.J., Randall, L., Poddubskaya, E.V., Scambia, G., Shparyk, Y.V., Lim, M.C., et al. (2021). Chemotherapy with or without avelumab followed by avelumab maintenance versus chemotherapy alone in patients with previously untreated epithelial ovarian cancer (JAVELIN Ovarian 100): an open-label, randomised, phase 3 trial. Lancet Oncol 22, 1275–1289. 10.1016/S1470–2045(21)00342-9.

Moore, K., Colombo, N., Scambia, G., Kim, B.G., Oaknin, A., Friedlander, M., Lisyanskaya, A., Floquet, A., Leary, A., Sonke, G.S., et al. (2018). Maintenance olaparib in patients with newly diagnosed advanced ovarian cancer. N Engl J Med 379, 2495–2505. 10.1056/NEJMoa1810858.

Moore, K.N., Bookman, M., Sehouli, J., Miller, A., Anderson, C., Scambia, G., Myers, T., Taskiran, C., Robison, K., Mäenpää, J., et al. (2021a). Atezolizumab, bevacizumab, and chemotherapy for newly diagnosed stage III or IV ovarian cancer: placebo-controlled randomized phase III trial (IMagyn050/GOG 3015/ENGOT-OV39). J Clin Oncol 39, 1842–1855. 10.1200/jco.21.00306.

Moore, K.N., Oza, A.M., Colombo, N., Oaknin, A., Scambia, G., Lorusso, D., Konecny, G.E., Banerjee, S., Murphy, C.G., Tanyi, J.L., et al. (2021b). Phase III, randomized trial of mirvetuximab soravtansine versus chemotherapy in patients with platinum-resistant ovarian cancer: primary analysis of FORWARD I. Ann Oncol *32*, 757–765. 10.1016/j. annonc.2021.02.017.

Moore, K.N., Secord, A.A., Geller, M.A., Miller, D.S., Cloven, N., Fleming, G.F., Wahner Hendrickson, A.E., Azodi, M., DiSilvestro, P., Oza, A.M., et al. (2019). Niraparib monotherapy for late-line treatment of ovarian cancer (QUADRA): a multicentre, open-label, single-arm, phase 2 trial. Lancet Oncol. 10.1016/S1470-2045(19)30029-4.

Muggia, F.M., Braly, P.S., Brady, M.F., Sutton, G., Niemann, T.H., Lentz, S.L., Alvarez, R.D., Kucera, P.R., and Small, J.M. (2000). Phase III randomized study of cisplatin versus paclitaxel versus cisplatin and paclitaxel in patients with suboptimal stage III or IV ovarian cancer: a Gynecologic Oncology Group study. J Clin Oncol *18*, 106–115. 10.1200/JCO.2000.18.1.106.

Oza, A.M., Cook, A.D., Pfisterer, J., Embleton, A., Ledermann, J.A., Pujade-Lauraine, E., Kristensen, G., Carey, M.S., Beale, P., Cervantes, A., et al. (2015). Standard chemotherapy with or without bevacizumab for women with newly diagnosed ovarian cancer (ICON7): overall survival results of a phase 3 randomised trial. Lancet Oncol *16*, 928–936. 10.1016/S1470-2045(15)00086-8.

Ozols, R.F., Bundy, B.N., Greer, B.E., Fowler, J.M., Clarke-Pearson, D., Burger, R.A., Mannel, R.S., DeGeest, K., Hartenbach, E.M., Baergen, R., and Gynecologic Oncology Group. (2003). Phase III trial of carboplatin and paclitaxel compared with cisplatin and paclitaxel in patients with optimally resected stage III ovarian cancer: a Gynecologic Oncology Group study. J Clin Oncol *21*, 3194–3200. 10.1200/JCO.2003.02.153.

Panici, P.B., Maggioni, A., Hacker, N., Landoni, F., Ackermann, S., Campagnutta, E., Tamussino, K., Winter, R., Pellegrino, A., Greggi, S., et al. (2005). Systematic aortic and pelvic lymphadenectomy versus resection of bulky nodes only in optimally debulked advanced ovarian cancer: a randomized clinical trial. J Natl Cancer Inst *97*, 560–566. 10.1093/jnci/dji102.

Parmar, M.K., Ledermann, J.A., Colombo, N., du Bois, A., Delaloye, J.F., Kristensen, G.B., Wheeler, S., Swart, A.M., Qian, W., Torri, V., et al. (2003). Paclitaxel plus platinum-based chemotherapy versus conventional platinum-based chemotherapy in women with relapsed ovarian cancer: the ICON4/AGO-OVAR-2.2 trial. Lancet *361*, 2099–2106.

Perren, T.J., Swart, A.M., Pfisterer, J., Ledermann, J.A., Pujade-Lauraine, E., Kristensen, G., Carey, M.S., Beale, P., Cervantes, A., Kurzeder, C., et al. (2011). A phase 3 trial of bevacizumab in ovarian cancer. N Engl J Med *365*, 2484–2496. 10.1056/NEJMoa1103799.

Petrillo, M., Vizzielli, G., Fanfani, F., Gallotta, V., Cosentino, F., Chiantera, V., Legge, F., Carbone, V., Scambia, G., and Fagotti, A. (2015). Definition of a dynamic laparoscopic model for the prediction of incomplete cytoreduction in advanced epithelial ovarian cancer: proof of a concept. Gynecol Oncol *139*, 5–9. 10.1016/j.ygyno.2015.07.095.

Pfisterer, J., Joly, F., Kristensen, G., Rau, J., Mahner, S., Pautier, P., El-Balat, A., Kurtz, J.E., Canzler, U., Sehouli, J., et al. (2021). Optimal treatment duration of bevacizumab (BEV) combined with carboplatin and paclitaxel in patients (pts) with primary epithelial ovarian (EOC), fallopian tube (FTC) or peritoneal cancer (PPC): a multicenter open-label randomized 2-arm phase 3 ENGOT/GCIG trial of the AGO Study Group, GINECO, and NSGO (AGO-OVAR 17/BOOST, GINECO OV118, ENGOT Ov-15, NCT01462890). J Clin Oncol *39*, 5501–5501. 10.1200/JCO.2021.39.15_suppl.5501.

Pfisterer, J., Plante, M., Vergote, I., du Bois, A., Hirte, H., Lacave, A.J., Wagner, U., Stahle, A., Stuart, G., Kimmig, R., et al. (2006). Gemcitabine plus carboplatin compared with carboplatin in patients with platinum-sensitive recurrent ovarian cancer: an intergroup trial of the AGO-OVAR, the NCIC CTG, and the EORTC GCG. J Clin Oncol *24*, 4699–4707. 10.1200/JCO.2006.06.0913.

Pfisterer, J., Shannon, C.M., Baumann, K., Rau, J., Harter, P., Joly, F., Sehouli, J., Canzler, U., Schmalfeldt, B., Dean, A.P., et al. (2020). Bevacizumab and platinum-based combinations for recurrent ovarian cancer: a randomised, open-label, phase 3 trial. Lancet Oncol *21*, 699–709. 10.1016/S1470–2045(20)30142-X.

Piccart, M.J., Bertelsen, K., James, K., Cassidy, J., Mangioni, C., Simonsen, E., Stuart, G., Kaye, S., Vergote, I., Blom, R., et al. (2000). Randomized intergroup trial of cisplatin-paclitaxel versus cisplatin-cyclophosphamide in women with advanced epithelial ovarian cancer: three-year results. J Natl Cancer Inst *92*, 699–708.

Pignata, S., Lorusso, D., Joly, F., Gallo, C., Colombo, N., Sessa, C., Bamias, A., Salutari, V., Selle, F., Frezzini, S., et al. (2021). Carboplatin-based doublet plus bevacizumab beyond progression versus carboplatin-based doublet alone in patients with platinum-sensitive ovarian cancer: a randomised, phase 3 trial. Lancet Oncol 22, 267–276. 10.1016/S1470–2045(20)30637-9.

Pignata, S., Scambia, G., Ferrandina, G., Savarese, A., Sorio, R., Breda, E., Gebbia, V., Musso, P., Frigerio, L., Del Medico, P., et al. (2011). Carboplatin plus paclitaxel versus carboplatin plus pegylated liposomal doxorubicin as first-line treatment for patients with ovarian cancer: the MITO-2 randomized phase III trial. J Clin Oncol *29*, 3628–3635. 10.1200/JCO.2010.33.8566.

Pignata, S., Scambia, G., Katsaros, D., Gallo, C., Pujade-Lauraine, E., De Placido, S., Bologna, A., Weber, B., Raspagliesi, F., Panici, P.B., et al. (2014). Carboplatin plus paclitaxel once a week versus every 3 weeks in patients with advanced ovarian cancer (MITO-7): a randomised, multicentre, open-label, phase 3 trial. Lancet Oncol *15*, 396–405. 10.1016/S1470–2045(14)70049-X.

Poveda, A., Floquet, A., Ledermann, J.A., Asher, R., Penson, R.T., Oza, A.M., Korach, J., Huzarski, T., Pignata, S., Friedlander, M., et al. (2021). Olaparib tablets as maintenance therapy in patients with platinum-sensitive relapsed ovarian cancer and a BRCA1/2 mutation (SOLO2/ENGOT-Ov21): a final analysis of a double-blind, randomised, placebo-controlled, phase 3 trial. Lancet Oncol *22*, 620–631. 10.1016/S1470-2045(21)00073-5.

Poveda, A.M., Selle, F., Hilpert, F., Reuss, A., Savarese, A., Vergote, I., Witteveen, P., Bamias, A., Scotto, N., Mitchell, L., and Pujade-Lauraine, E. (2015). Bevacizumab combined with weekly paclitaxel, pegylated liposomal doxorubicin, or topotecan in platinum-resistant recurrent ovarian cancer: analysis by chemotherapy cohort of the randomized phase III AURELIA trial. J Clin Oncol *33*, 3836–3838. 10.1200/JCO.2015.63.1408.

Pujade-Lauraine, E., Hilpert, F., Weber, B., Reuss, A., Poveda, A., Kristensen, G., Sorio, R., Vergote, I., Witteveen, P., Bamias, A., et al. (2014). Bevacizumab combined with chemotherapy for platinum-resistant recurrent ovarian cancer: the AURELIA open-label randomized phase III trial. J Clin Oncol *32*, 1302–1308. 10.1200/JCO.2013.51.4489.

Pujade-Lauraine, E., Ledermann, J.A., Selle, F., Gebski, V., Penson, R.T., Oza, A.M., Korach, J., Huzarski, T., Poveda, A., Pignata, S., et al. (2017). Olaparib tablets as maintenance therapy in patients with platinum-sensitive, relapsed ovarian cancer and a BRCA1/2 mutation (SOLO2/ENGOT-Ov21): a double-blind, randomised, placebo-controlled, phase 3 trial. Lancet Oncol *18*, 1274–1284. 10.1016/S1470-2045(17)30469-2.

Pujade-Lauraine, E., Selle, F., Scambia, G., Asselain, B., Marmé, F., Lindemann, K., Colombo, N., Madry, R., Glasspool, R., M., Dubot, C., Oaknin, A., Zamagni, C., Heitz, F., Gladieff, L., Rubio-Pérez, M.J., Scollo, P., Blakeley, C., Shaw, B., Ray-Coquard, I.L., and Redondo, A. (2021). Maintenance olaparib rechallenge in patients (pts) with ovarian carcinoma (OC) previously treated with a PARP inhibitor (PARPi): phase IIIb OReO/ENGOT Ov-38 trial. ESMO. Ann Oncology *32*, S1308–1309.

Pujade-Lauraine, E., Wagner, U., Aavall-Lundqvist, E., Gebski, V., Heywood, M., Vasey, P.A., Volgger, B., Vergote, I., Pignata, S., Ferrero, A., et al. (2010). Pegylated liposomal doxorubicin and carboplatin compared with paclitaxel and carboplatin for patients with platinum-sensitive ovarian cancer in late relapse. J Clin Oncol *28*, 3323–3329. 10.1200/ JCO.2009.25.7519.

Ray-Coquard, I., Pautier, P., Pignata, S., Perol, D., Gonzalez-Martin, A., Berger, R., Fujiwara, K., Vergote, I., Colombo, N., Maenpaa, J., et al. (2019). Olaparib plus bevacizumab as first-line maintenance in ovarian cancer. N Engl J Med *381*, 2416–2428. 10.1056/NEJMoa1911361.

Rustin, G.J., van der Burg, M.E., Griffin, C.L., Guthrie, D., Lamont, A., Jayson, G.C., Kristensen, G., Mediola, C., Coens, C., Qian, W., et al. (2010). Early versus delayed treatment of relapsed ovarian cancer (MRC OV05/EORTC 55955): a randomised trial. Lancet *376*, 1155–1163. 10.1016/S0140-6736(10)61268-8.

Salani, R., Santillan, A., Zahurak, M.L., Giuntoli, R.L., 2nd, Gardner, G.J., Armstrong, D.K., and Bristow, R.E. (2007). Secondary cytoreductive surgery for localized, recurrent epithelial ovarian cancer: analysis of prognostic factors and survival outcome. Cancer *109*, 685–691. 10.1002/cncr.22447.

Schmeler, K.M., Tao, X., Frumovitz, M., Deavers, M.T., Sun, C.C., Sood, A.K., Brown, J., Gershenson, D.M., and Ramirez, P.T. (2010). Prevalence of lymph node metastasis in primary mucinous carcinoma of the ovary. Obstet Gynecol *116*, 269–273. 10.1097/ AOG.0b013e3181e7961d.

Senekjian, E.K., Weiser, P.A., Talerman, A., and Herbst, A.L. (1989). Vinblastine, cisplatin, cyclophosphamide, bleomycin, doxorubicin, and etoposide in the treatment of small cell carcinoma of the ovary. Cancer *64*, 1183–1187. 10.1002/1097-0142(19890915)64: 6<1183::aid-cncr2820640603>3.0.co;2-n.

Shi, T., Zhu, J., Feng, Y., Tu, D., Zhang, Y., Zhang, P., Jia, H., Huang, X., Cai, Y., Yin, S., et al. (2021). Secondary cytoreduction followed by chemotherapy versus chemotherapy alone in platinum-sensitive relapsed ovarian cancer (SOC-1): a multicentre, open-label, randomised, phase 3 trial. Lancet Oncol *22*, 439–449. 10.1016/S1470-2045(21)00006-1.

Suidan, R.S., Ramirez, P.T., Sarasohn, D.M., Teitcher, J.B., Mironov, S., Iyer, R.B., Zhou, Q., Iasonos, A., Paul, H., Hosaka, M., et al. (2014). A multicenter prospective trial evaluating the ability of preoperative computed tomography scan and serum CA-125 to predict suboptimal cytoreduction at primary debulking surgery for advanced ovarian, fallopian tube, and peritoneal cancer. Gynecol Oncol *134*, 455–461. 10.1016/j.ygyno.2014.07.002.

Swisher, E.M., Lin, K.K., Oza, A.M., Scott, C.L., Giordano, H., Sun, J., Konecny, G.E., Coleman, R.L., Tinker, A.V., O'Malley, D.M., et al. (2017). Rucaparib in relapsed, platinum-sensitive high-grade ovarian carcinoma (ARIEL2 Part 1): an international, multicentre, open-label, phase 2 trial. Lancet Oncol *18*, 75–87. 10.1016/S1470-2045(16)30559-9.

Trimbos, J.B., Parmar, M., Vergote, I., Guthrie, D., Bolis, G., Colombo, N., Vermorken, J.B., Torri, V., Mangioni, C., Pecorelli, S., et al. (2003a). International Collaborative Ovarian Neoplasm trial 1 and adjuvant chemotherapy in ovarian neoplasm trial: two parallel randomized phase III trials of adjuvant chemotherapy in patients with early-stage ovarian carcinoma. J Natl Cancer Inst *95*, 105–112.

Trimbos, J.B., Vergote, I., Bolis, G., Vermorken, J.B., Mangioni, C., Madronal, C., Franchi, M., Tateo, S., Zanetta, G., Scarfone, G., et al. (2003b). Impact of adjuvant chemotherapy and surgical staging in early-stage ovarian carcinoma: European Organisation for Research and Treatment of Cancer-Adjuvant Chemotherapy in Ovarian Neoplasm trial. J Natl Cancer Inst *95*, 113–125.

van Driel, W.J., Koole, S.N., Sikorska, K., Schagen van Leeuwen, J.H., Schreuder, H.W.R., Hermans, R.H.M., de Hingh, I., van der Velden, J., Arts, H.J., Massuger, L., et al. (2018). Hyperthermic intraperitoneal chemotherapy in ovarian cancer. N Engl J Med *378*, 230–240. 10.1056/NEJMoa1708618.

Vergote, I., Coens, C., Nankivell, M., Kristensen, G.B., Parmar, M.K.B., Ehlen, T., Jayson, G.C., Johnson, N., Swart, A.M., Verheijen, R., et al. (2018). Neoadjuvant chemotherapy versus debulking surgery in advanced tubo-ovarian cancers: pooled analysis of individual patient data from the EORTC 55971 and CHORUS trials. Lancet Oncol 19, 1680–1687. 10.1016/S1470-2045(18)30566-7.

Vergote, I., Trope, C.G., Amant, F., Kristensen, G.B., Ehlen, T., Johnson, N., Verheijen, R.H., van der Burg, M.E., Lacave, A.J., Panici, P.B., et al. (2010). Neoadjuvant chemotherapy or primary surgery in stage IIIC or IV ovarian cancer. N Engl J Med 363, 943–953. 10.1056/NEJMoa0908806.

Wagner, U., Marth, C., Largillier, R., Kaern, J., Brown, C., Heywood, M., Bonaventura, T., Vergote, I., Piccirillo, M.C., Fossati, R., et al. (2012). Final overall survival results of phase III GCIG CALYPSO trial of pegylated liposomal doxorubicin and carboplatin vs paclitaxel and carboplatin in platinum-sensitive ovarian cancer patients. Br J Cancer 107, 588–591. 10.1038/bjc.2012.307.

Walker, J.L., Brady, M.F., Wenzel, L., Fleming, G.F., Huang, H.Q., DiSilvestro, P.A., Fujiwara, K., Alberts, D.S., Zheng, W., Tewari, K.S., et al. (2019). Randomized trial of intravenous versus intraperitoneal chemotherapy plus bevacizumab in advanced ovarian carcinoma: an NRG oncology/Gynecologic Oncology Group study. J Clin Oncol 37, 1380–1390. 10.1200/JCO.18.01568.

Williams, S., Blessing, J.A., Liao, S.Y., Ball, H., and Hanjani, P. (1994). Adjuvant therapy of ovarian germ cell tumors with cisplatin, etoposide, and bleomycin: a trial of the Gynecologic Oncology Group. J Clin Oncol 12, 701–706. 10.1200/JCO.1994.12.4.701.

Williams, S.D., Blessing, J.A., Moore, D.H., Homesley, H.D., and Adcock, L. (1989). Cisplatin, vinblastine, and bleomycin in advanced and recurrent ovarian germ-cell tumors. A trial of the Gynecologic Oncology Group. Ann Intern Med 111, 22–27.

Zamarin, D., Burger, R.A., Sill, M.W., Powell, D.J., Jr., Lankes, H.A., Feldman, M.D., Zivanovic, O., Gunderson, C., Ko, E., Mathews, C., et al. (2020). Randomized phase II trial of nivolumab versus nivolumab and ipilimumab for recurrent or persistent ovarian cancer: an NRG oncology study. J Clin Oncol 38, 1814–1823. 10.1200/JCO.19.02059.

Zivanovic, O., Chi, D.S., Zhou, Q., Iasonos, A., Konner, J.A., Makker, V., Grisham, R.N., Brown, A.K., Nerenstone, S., Diaz, J.P., et al. (2021). Secondary cytoreduction and carboplatin hyperthermic intraperitoneal chemotherapy for platinum-sensitive recurrent ovarian cancer: an MSK team ovary phase II study. J Clin Oncol 39, 2594–2604. 10.1200/JCO.21.00605.

Zsiros, E., Lynam, S., Attwood, K.M., Wang, C., Chilakapati, S., Gomez, E.C., Liu, S., Akers, S., Lele, S., Frederick, P.J., and Odunsi, K. (2021). Efficacy and safety of pembrolizumab in combination with bevacizumab and oral metronomic cyclophosphamide in the treatment of recurrent ovarian cancer: a phase 2 nonrandomized clinical trial. JAMA Oncol 7, 78–85. 10.1001/jamaoncol.2020.5945.

Cervical Cancer 3

3.1 STUDIES ADDRESSING SURGICAL TREATMENT

Study: GOG 49

- **Citation:** (Delgado et al., 1989)
- **Highlight:** Prognostic factors for microscopic PLN involvement
- **Design:**
  - 645 patients with primary stage I squamous cell carcinoma >3 mm invasion without gross disease beyond cervix/uterus and with negative PALN s/p radical hysterectomy and PLND
- **Results:**
  - Risk factors for microscopic PLN metastasis
    - Depth of stromal invasion (p = 0.001)
      - Absolute dimension: 3.4% vs. 15.1% vs. 22.2% vs. 38.8% vs. 22.6% (≤5 mm vs. 6–10 mm vs. 11–15 mm vs. 16–20 mm vs. ≥21 mm)
      - Fractions: 4.5% vs. 13.3% vs. 26.4% (superficial vs. middle vs. deep third)
    - Gross primary tumor
      - 8.9% vs. 20.9% (p = 0.009) (occult vs. gross)
    - Capillary lymphatic space (CLS) invasion
      - 8.2% vs. 25.4% (negative vs. positive)
    - Tumor grade: 9.7%, 13.9%, and 21.8% for G1, G2, and G3 (p = 0.01)
    - Parametrial status: 13.5% vs. 43.2% (p = 0.0001)
  - Not statistically significant: Age, surgical margins (15.2% vs. 25% for the 20 patients with positive margins, i.e., non-significance may be due to small number), performance status, tumor diameter (in cm), tumor description (e.g., exophytic), quadrant involvement, and keratinizing status of tumor cells
  - Independent risk factors on multivariate analysis
    - CLS (p < 0.0001)
    - Depth of invasion (p < 0.0001)
    - Parametrial involvement (p = 0.0005)
    - Age (p = 0.02)

DOI: 10.1201/9781003229711-3

Study: GOG 49

- **Citation:** (Delgado et al., 1990)
- **Highlight:** Prognostic factors for DFI
- **Results:**
  - 3-yr DFI
    - Pelvic LNs
      - 85.6% vs. 74.4% (545 patients with negative PLNs vs. 100 patients with positive PLNs)
      - No correlation of large number of positive PLNs with prognosis: 72.1% vs. 86.4% vs. 64.6% (1 vs. 2 vs. ≥3 positive PLNs)
    - Depth of stromal invasion
      - Absolute dimension: 94.6% vs. 86% vs. 75.2% vs. 71.5% vs. 59.5% (≤5 vs. 6–10 vs. 11–15 vs. 16–20 vs. ≥21 mm)
      - Fractions: 94.1% vs. 84.5% vs. 73.6% (superficial vs. middle vs. deep third)
    - Clinical tumor size
      - 94.8% vs. 88.1% vs. 67.6% (occult vs. ≤3 cm vs. >3 cm)
    - CLS invasion
      - 88.9% vs. 77% (negative vs. positive)
    - Tumor grade: 90.6%, 86%, and 76% for G1, G2, and G3 (p = 0.001)
    - Parametrial status: 84.9% vs. 69.6% (p = 0.03)
    - No difference for
      - Age, surgical margins (3-yr DFI 84.3% vs. 69.1% for the 20 patients with positive margins, i.e., non-significance may be due to small number), tumor description (e.g., exophytic), quadrant involvement, and keratinizing status of tumor cells
- **Conclusion:**
  - → Clinical tumor size, CLS, and depth of tumor invasion independent prognostic factors (identified using proportional hazard model)

Study: Landoni study

- **Citation:** (Landoni et al., 1997)
- **Highlight:** Radical hysterectomy vs. radical radiation
- **Design:**
  - 343 patients with stage IB (1 and 2) and IIA cervical cancer randomized to radical hysterectomy vs. radical RT
  - Radical RT: EBRT with median total dose of 47 Gy, 1.8–2.0 Gy fractions over 4–5 wks; after 2 wks, LDR BCT; total dose at point A 70–90 Gy; at point B >50 Gy; if necessary, parametrial boost; when lymphangiography showed common iliac or para-aortic metastases, PALNs treated with 45 Gy over 5 wks with additional boost to positive nodes
  - Radical surgery (radical hysterectomy): Class III abdominal hysterectomy and PLND; if age <40 and squamous cell carcinoma, one ovary preserved and suspended

- Number of patients with tumor ≤4 cm/>4 cm similar in both groups: 115/55 in surgery and 113/54 in the RT group
- Adjuvant RT after surgery if
  - pT2b or greater
  - <3 mm of safe cervical stroma
  - Cut-through
  - Positive PLNs
- Adjuvant RT: EBRT in 1.8–2.0 Gy fractions qd, over 5–6 wks, total of 50.4 Gy; if surgical specimen shows metastasis in common iliac or para-aortic nodes with dose of 45 Gy over 5 wks

- **Results:**
  - Median follow-up: 87 months
  - 5-yr PFS for both groups: 74%
  - 5-yr OS for both groups: 83%
    - 5-yr OS stratified by cervical diameter similar
      - ≤4 cm: 87% vs. 90% (surgery vs. RT)
      - >4 cm: 70% vs. 72%
    - 5-yr OS stratified by histology
      - For squamous cell carcinoma: 80% vs. 82%
      - For adenocarcinoma: 70% vs. 59% (p = 0.05) (5-yr PFS: 66% vs. 47%; p = 0.02)
  - Recurrences in 25% vs. 26% (surgery vs. RT)
  - Risk factors in univariate and multivariate analyses
    - Cervical diameter
    - Positive lymphangiography
    - Adenocarcinoma histology
  - Severe morbidity: 28% vs. 12% (surgery vs. RT) (p = 0.0004)
    - Short-term complications: 16% vs. 20% vs. 7% (surgery, surgery + RT, and RT alone)
    - Long-term complications: 24% vs. 29% vs. 16%
- **Conclusion:**
  - → There is no treatment of choice for early-stage cervical cancer; combination of surgery and RT has worst morbidity (especially urological complications)

Study: GOG 71

- **Citation:** (Keys et al., 2003)
- **Highlight:** RT ± extrafascial hysterectomy (initially joint by RTOG 84–12)
- **Background:**
  - Case series from MD Anderson in 1960s and 1970s suggested that bulky tumors better addressed by radical hysterectomy than by additional intracavitary radiation, and radical hysterectomy reduced risk of central failure; other centers reported that size, not barrel shape, the principal factor for decreasing local control

- **Design:**
  - 256 patients with stage IB2 (bulky IB *or* exophytic or 'barrel'-shaped tumors ≥4 cm) randomized to external and intracavitary radiation (RT) vs. attenuated irradiation followed by extrafascial hysterectomy (RT + HYST)
  - External RT with total dose of 40 Gy (RT group) and 45 Gy (RT + HYST group)
  - Intracavitary radiation 1–2 wks after completion of EBRT
    - 40 Gy to point A (2 cm lateral and 2 cm superior to cervical os) (group RT); 30 Gy to point A (RT + HYST group)
    - Minimum dose of 55 Gy to point B for both groups
    - No interstitial RT
  - Hysterectomy 2–6 wks after completion of RT
- **Results:**
  - 25% of patients with tumors ≥7 cm
  - Identified prognostic factors
    - Tumor size (most pronounced)
    - GOG (Zubrod) performance status 2
    - Age
  - RT + HYST: No increase in grade 3 and 4 AE (10% in both)
  - Lower cumulative incidence of local relapse in RT + HYST (at 5 yrs: 27% vs. 14%)
  - No statistical difference in outcomes
    - Progression: RR 0.77 (RT + HYST) (p = 0.07); median PFS for RT 7.4 yrs; for RT + HYST not reached (PFS 53% at 8.4 yrs)
    - Disease-related deaths in 35% vs. 34% (RT vs. RT + HYST)
    - Death: RR 0.89 (p = 0.26)
- **Conclusion:**
  - → No clinical benefit of extrafascial hysterectomy; however, patients with 4, 5, and 6 cm tumors may have benefitted from hysterectomy

Study: LACC trial (Laparoscopic Approach to Cervical Cancer)

- **Citation:** (Ramirez et al., 2018)
- **Highlight:** Minimally invasive vs. open radical hysterectomy
- **Design:**
  - Non-inferior trial including 631 patients with stage IA1 (with LVSI), IA2, IB1 cervical cancer (squamous cell carcinoma, adenocarcinoma, and adeno-squamous carcinoma) randomized to minimally invasive vs. open surgery
- **Results:**
  - 84.4% laparoscopy and 15.6% robot-assisted surgery
  - Mean age: 46.0
  - 91.9% with stage IB1
  - Groups similar in histologic subtype, LN involvement, tumor size, grade, and rate of adjuvant therapy
  - 4.5-yr DFS: 86.0% vs. 96.5% (minimally invasive vs. open)

- 3-yr DFS: 91.2% vs. 97.1% (HR for disease recurrence or death 3.74 [CI = 1.63–8.58])
- Difference remained after adjustment for age, BMI, stage, lymphovascular invasion, and LN involvement
- 3-yr OS: 93.8% vs. 99.0% (HR for death from any cause 6.00 [CI = 1.77–20.30])
- **Conclusion:**
  - → In this trial, minimally invasive radical hysterectomy with lower DFS and OS than open radical hysterectomy

Study: LACC trial

- **Citation:** (Frumovitz et al., 2020)
- **Highlight:** Quality of life for minimally invasive vs. open radical hysterectomy
- **Design:**
  - Functional Assessment of Cancer Therapy—Cervical (FACT-Cx)
- **Results:**
  - Median follow-up: 3 yrs
  - No differences in the FACT-Cx total scores at baseline before surgery, 6 wks after surgery, or 3 months after surgery
- **Conclusion:**
  - Postoperative quality of life is similar between treatment groups

3.2 STUDIES ADDRESSING ADJUVANT THERAPY

Study: GOG 92

- **Citation:** (Sedlis et al., 1999)
- **Highlight:** Early-stage intermediate risk; adjuvant RT = Sedlis criteria
- **Design:**
  - 277 patients with stage IB cervical cancer s/p RH and PLND with at least two of the following risk factors: >1/3 stromal invasion, CLS involvement, and large clinical tumor diameter randomized to pelvic RT vs. NFT
    - Eligibility criteria (based on GOG 49 [Delgado et al., 1989])

CLS	STROMAL INVASION	TUMOR SIZE (cm)
+	Deep 1/3	Any
+	Middle 1/3	≥ 2
+	Superficial 1/3	≥ 5
−	Deep or middle 1/3	≥ 4

- RT started within 4–6 wks postoperatively
  - EBRT: No BCT
  - 46 Gy in 23 fractions to 50.4 Gy in 28 fractions (five fractions/wk → daily dose of 1.8–2.0 Gy over 4.5–6 wks); break only allowed for up to 1 wk
- **Results:**
  - Overall recurrences: 15% (21 patients) vs. 28% (39 patients) (RT vs. NFT)
    - Vaginal/pelvic recurrences: 18% vs. 27%
    - RR for recurrence in RT group: 0.53 (p = 0.008)
    - 2-yr PFS: 97% vs. 88%
  - 18 patients (13%) died in RT group (15 of cancer) vs. 30 patients (21%) in NFT group (25 of cancer)
    - Relative mortality rate: 0.64 (i.e., indicating 36% less mortality in radiation group); significance not provided because data not mature
  - Grade 3 or 4 AEs
    - Urologic: 4 (3.1%) vs. 2 (1.4%)
    - Hematologic: 3 (2.3%) vs. 1 (0.7%)
    - Neurologic: 1 (0.8%) vs. 0
    - GI: None
- **Conclusion:**
  - → Adjuvant pelvic RT after radical surgery reduces recurrences at cost of grade 3 (6%) or 4 AEs (2.1%)

Study: GOG 92

- **Citation:** (Rotman et al., 2006)
- **Highlight:** Long-term follow-up
- **Results:**
  - Overall
    - 24 vs. 43 recurrences (RT vs. NFT)
    - HR for progression: 0.54 (CI = 0.35–0.81); p = 0.007
    - HR for progression or death: 0.58 (CI = 0.4–0.85); p = 0.009
  - For adenosquamous and adenocarcinoma
    - 8.8% (3/34) vs. 44% (11/25) recurred (HR 0.23 [CI: 0.07–0.74]; p = 0.019)
  - HR for death: 0.7 (CI = 0.45–1.05); p = 0.074
- **Conclusion:**
  - → Pelvic RT after radical surgery reduces risk of recurrence and prolongs PFS in stage IB cervical cancer but not OS
  - RT particularly beneficial in adenocarcinoma or adenosquamous

Study: GOG 109

- **Citation:** (Peters et al., 2000)
- **Highlight:** Early-stage high risk; CTRT

- **Design:**
  - 243 patients with stage IA2, IB, IIA s/p radical hysterectomy, and PLND with positive PLNs and/or positive margins and/or microscopic involvement of parametrium randomized to RT vs. RT + CT
  - EBRT in both groups: 49.3 Gy in 29 fractions
  - CT: Cisplatin 70 mg/m^2 and 96-hr infusion of 5 FU 1,000 mg/m^2/d q 3 wks × 4 C, with first and second cycles given concurrent to RT (and third and fourth 'adjuvant')
- **Results:**
  - 4-yr PFS: 63% vs. 80% (RT vs. RT + CT) (HR = 2.01; p = 0.003)
  - In the RT group, patients with adenocarcinoma or adenosquamous carcinoma with worse prognosis than squamous cell carcinoma; addition of CT makes this difference in the RT–CT group disappear
  - 4-yr OS: 71% vs. 81% (HR = 1.96; p = 0.007)
  - Grade 3 and 4 hematologic and GI toxicity more frequent in the RT + CT group
- **Conclusion:**
  - → Addition of cisplatin-based CT to RT improves PFS and OS compared to RT in high-risk early-stage patients undergoing radical hysterectomy and PLND

Study: GOG 274, RTOG 07–24 (Outback trial)

- **Citation:** NCT00980954, ongoing, presented at ASCO 2021 (Mileshkin et al., 2021)
- **Highlight:** Early-stage high-risk cervical cancer
- **Design:**
  - CT and pelvic RT with and without additional adjuvant CT for high-risk early stage (IA2, IB, and IIA) cervical cancer after radical hysterectomy and PLND
    - Any of the following
      - Positive PLN
      - Positive parametrium
      - Positive PALN that has been completely resected and is PET/CT negative (PET only required if positive PALN during surgery)
  - Arm I (co)
    - EBRT or IMRT to pelvis qd for 5 d a week for 5–6 wks; concurrent cisplatin iv over 1 hr q wk × 6 C
  - Arm II (ACT):
    - CTRT as in arm I; 4–6 wks after CTRT, carboplatin iv over 30 min and paclitaxel iv over 3 hrs on day 1; q 3 wks × 4 C
- **Results:**
  - Median follow-up: 60 months
  - 5-yr OS: 72% vs. 71% (HR 0.91 [CI = 0.7–1.18] (ACT vs. co)
  - 5-yr PFS: 63% vs. 61% (HR 0.87 [CI = 0.7–1.08])

- Patterns of disease recurrence similar in the two groups
- ≥ Grade 3 AE: 81% vs. 62%
- **Conclusion:**
  - → Adjuvant CT after standard cis-RT in locally advanced cervical cancer did not improve OS or PFS

3.3 STUDIES ADDRESSING PRIMARY CHEMORADIATION THERAPY

Study: GOG 123: Keys trial

- **Citation:** (Keys et al., 1999)
- **Highlight:** Bulky IB
- **Design:**
  - 369 patients with bulky stage IB (≥4 cm) cervical cancer and negative LNs (on imaging or biopsy) randomized to RT vs. CTRT followed by hysterectomy for both groups
  - RT
    - EBRT: 45 Gy in 20 fractions, followed by LDR ICBT of 30 Gy to point A; 55 Gy to point B
  - CT
    - Cisplatin: 40 mg/m^2 q wk × 6 C (given during EBRT)
  - Total extrafascial hysterectomy followed completion of RT by 3–6 wks
    - 168/186 in the RT group and 174/183 in the CTRT group underwent hysterectomy
- **Results:**
  - Grade 3 or 4 hematologic AE: 21% vs. 2% (CTRT vs. RT)
  - GI AE, mostly mild: 14% vs. 5%
  - Median follow-up: 36 months
  - RR for progression: 0.51 favoring CTRT
  - 3-yr PFS: 79% vs. 63% (p < 0.001) (CTRT vs. RT)
  - 3-yr OS: 83% vs. 74% (p = 0.008)
- **Conclusion:**
  - → Adding weekly cisplatin to pelvic RT followed by hysterectomy reduces risk of recurrence and death in bulky IB cervical cancer
  - Based on GOG 71, elimination of hysterectomy would not have affected increase in survival; hence, RT with cisplatin should be adequate for bulky stage IB

Study: GOG 123: Keys trial

- **Citation:** (Stehman et al., 2007)
- **Highlight:** Long-term follow-up

- **Results:**
  - Median follow-up: 101 months
  - 6-yr PFS: 71% vs. 60% (CTRT vs. RT) (RR = 0.61 [CI: 0.43–0.85]; p < 0.004
  - 6-yr OS: 78% vs. 64% (RR = 0.63 [CI: 0.43–0.91]; p < 0.015
  - Overall late AE uncommon and no difference in rate
- **Conclusion:**
  - → Concurrent weekly cisplatin with RT improves long-term PFS and OS when compared with RT alone; the inclusion of hysterectomy has been discontinued on the basis of GOG 71; pending further trials: CisRT = standard against which other regimens should be compared

Study: RTOG 79-20

- **Citation:** (Rotman et al., 1990)
- **Highlight:** Extended field radiation therapy (EFRT)
- **Design:**
  - 367 patients with stage IB and IIA ≥4 cm, stage IIB without curative surgery, and no clinically apparent or surgically involved PALNs randomized to pelvic vs. pelvic plus para-aortic irradiation
  - Pelvic RT: 1.6–1.8 Gy qd for 5 d per week to 40–50 Gy total, completed in 4.5–6.5 wks
  - Para-aortic RT: 1.6–1.8 Gy qd for 5 d per week to 44–45 Gy total, completed in 4.5–5.5 wks
  - ICBT: Total of 30–40 Gy to point A
  - Stratified before randomization by histology, PALN status (negative vs. unevaluated), and stage
- **Results:**
  - Toxicities
    - − ≥ Grade 3 AE: 8% vs. 8% (pelvic vs. pelvic plus PA)
    - − In patients with prior abdominal surgery, pelvic plus para-aortic RT with more grade 4 and 5 AEs (2% vs. 11%)
  - 5-yr locoregional control: 66% vs. 75% (p = 0.21)
  - 5-yr distant metastasis: 32% vs. 25% (p = 0.17)
  - More patients fail first distally when treated only with pelvic RT (p = 0.04)
  - 5-yr OS: 55% vs. 65% (p = 0.043)
- **Conclusion:**
  - → Prophylactic treatment of PA LN had statistically significant survival benefit in early cervical cancer; trend also in NED survival and distant metastases

Study: RTOG 79-20

- **Citation:** (Rotman et al., 1995)
- **Highlight:** Long-term follow-up

- **Results:**
  - 10-yr OS: 44% vs. 55% (p = 0.02) (pelvic vs. pelvic plus PA)
  - 10-yr PFS: 40% vs. 42%
    - Locoregional failures: 35% vs. 31%
    - Cumulative incidence for distant failure lower in pelvic plus PA (p = 0.053)
    - Survival following first failure higher in pelvic plus PA (p = 0.007)
    - Higher percentage of local failures salvaged in pelvic plus PA arm vs. pelvic (25% vs. 8%)
  - Cumulative incidence of grade 4 and 5 toxicities at 10 yrs: 4% vs. 8% (pelvic vs. pelvic plus PA)
  - If prior abdominal surgery, incidence of grade 4 and 5 toxicities: 2% vs. 11%
- **Conclusion:**
  - → Statistically significant difference in 10-yr OS without difference in DFS can be explained by (1) lower incidence of distant failures and (2) better salvage who failed locally

Study: RTOG 90-01

- **Citation:** (Morris et al., 1999)
- **Highlight:** For locally advanced cervical cancer or positive PLNs, extended field radiation therapy (EFRT) vs. chemoradiation (CTRT)
- **Design:**
  - 403 patients with stages IIB to IVA cervical cancer with tumor diameter ≥5 cm, or positive PLNs randomized to EFRT vs. pelvic RT with concomitant fluorouracil and cisplatin (CTRT)
    - EBRT delivered AP/PA or four-field box technique at 4 MV photons
    - EFRT up to space between L1/L2
    - Total dose of EBRT: 45 Gy (same for EFRT), 1.8 Gy per fraction; BCT after EBRT with cumulative dose to point A (2 cm lateral and 2 cm superior to cervical os) of at least 85 Gy
    - Within 16 hrs after first radiation fraction CT administered: Cisplatin 75 mg/m^2 over 4 hrs followed by fluorouracil 4,000 mg/m^2 over 96 hrs; thus, administered during days 1 through 5 of RT, q 3 wks × 3 C
- **Results:**
  - Median follow-up: 43 months
  - Higher rate of reversible hematologic effects in CTRT; seriousness of side effects similar in both groups
  - 5-yr PFS: 40% vs. 67% (p < 0.001) (EFRT vs. CTRT)
    - Locoregional recurrences: 35% vs. 19% (p < 0.001)
    - Distant metastasis: 33% vs. 14% (p < 0.001)
  - 5-yr OS: 58% vs. 73% (p = 0.004)
- **Conclusion:**
  - → Addition of fluorouracil and cisplatin to EBRT and BCT improved survival in locally advanced cervical cancer

Study: RTOG 90-01

- **Citation:** (Eifel et al., 2004)
- **Highlight:** Long-term follow-up
- **Results:**
  - Median follow-up time for 228 surviving patients: 6.6 yrs
  - Rate of serious late complications similar in both groups
  - Overall reduction in disease recurrence: 51% for CTRT patients
    - 5-yr locoregional failure: 34% vs. 18% (p < 0.0001) (EFRT vs. CTRT)
    - 5-yr para-aortic failure: 4% vs. 7% (p = 0.15)
    - 5-yr distant metastasis: 31% vs. 18% (p = 0.0013)
  - 8-yr OS: 41% vs. 67% (p < 0.0001)
    - In stages IB to IIB, 5-yr OS: 55% vs. 79% (p < 0.0001) and DFS: 46% vs. 74% (p < 0.0001)
    - In stages III to IVA, DFS: 37% vs. 54% (p = 0.05) and trend toward better OS: 45% vs. 59% (p = 0.07)
- **Conclusion:**
  - → Addition of fluorouracil and cisplatin to RT significantly improved survival without increasing rate of late treatment-related side effects

Study: GOG 85, SWOG 8695

- **Citation:** (Whitney et al., 1999)
- **Highlight:** For locally advanced cervical cancer, CTRT with 5-FU and cisplatin vs. CTRT with hydroxyurea (HU)
- **Design:**
  - 368 patients with stage IIB, III, or IVA cervical cancer and negative PALN randomized to pelvic RT plus concurrent 5-fluorouracil 1,000 mg/m²/d on days 2, 3, 4, 5 and 30, 31, 32, 33 and cisplatin 50 mg/m² on days 1 and 29 (CF) vs. same pelvic RT plus oral hydroxyurea 80 mg/kg every Monday and Thursday or Tuesday and Friday (HU) during RT
  - EBRT in AP/PA or four-field box technique: 40.8 Gy in 24 fractions (IIB) or 51 Gy in 30 fractions (III and IVA), then BCT with 40 Gy (IIB) or 30 Gy (III and IV) to point A; if necessary, boost to point B to 55 Gy (IIB) or 60 Gy (III and IV); if solely EBRT, then 61.2 Gy
- **Results:**
  - Severe or life-threatening leukopenia: 4% vs. 24% (CF vs. HU)
  - 6-yr PFS: 57% vs. 47% (p = 0.023)
  - Sites of recurrence similar
  - 6-yr OS: 55% vs. 43% (p = 0.018)
- **Conclusion:**
  - → Combination of 5-FU and cisplatin with RT offers better PFS and OS than HU, with manageable toxicity

Study: GOG 120

- **Citation:** (Rose et al., 1999)
- **Highlight:** For locally advanced cervical cancer, 3 CT (RT) regimens
- **Design:**
  - 526 patients with stages IIB, III, and IVA cervical cancer without involvement of PALN randomized to three different CT regimens concurrent to RT
    - RT
      - EBRT to whole pelvis: 40.8 or 51.0 Gy in 24 or 30 fractions, respectively
      - Delivered AP/PA or four-field box technique (AP, PA, and two lateral fields) with at least 4 MV photons
      - Followed within 1–3 wks by ICBT with total dose delivered 40 Gy to stage IIB and 30 Gy to stage III or IVA; total dose to point A was 80.8 Gy in stage IIb and 81.0 in stage III or IVA; total dose to point B (pelvic sidewall) was 55.0 Gy for stage IIB and 60.0 Gy for stage III or IVA
      - If ICBT could not be given, additional EBRT for a total of 61.2 Gy (interstitial and HDR); BCT not allowed
      - RT duration: 10 wks
      - Withheld if leukocytes less than 2,000, or GI or GU toxicity for up to 1 wk
    - CT
      - Cisplatin: 40 mg/m^2 q wk × 6 wks (group 1)
      - Cisplatin, fluorouracil, and hydroxyurea (group 2)
        - 50 mg/m^2 Cis on days 1 and 29, followed by 4 g/m^2 FU as 96-hr infusion on days 1 and 29, and 2 g/m^2 hydroxyurea po q wk × 6 wks
      - Hydroxyurea: 3 g/m^2 po 2×/wk × 6 wks (group 3)
    - Laboratory requirements:
      - Leukocytes at least 3,000
      - Platelets at least 100,000
      - Creatinine no higher than 2 mg/dl
      - Adequate liver function
- **Results:**
  - Median follow-up: 35 months
  - Both groups with cisplatin had higher rate of PFS than hydroxyurea alone (p < 0.001)
    - RR for progression or death 0.57 (CI: 0.42–0.78) for group 1; 0.55 (CI: 0.4–0.75) for group 2 compared with group 3
  - OS higher in groups 1 and 2 than in 3
    - RR of death: 0.61 (CI: 0.44–0.85) for group 1; 0.58 (CI: 0.41–0.81)
- **Conclusion:**
  - → Regimens of RT + CT that contain cisplatin improve PFS and OS in locally advanced cervical cancer

Study: Cochrane meta-analysis

- **Citation:** (Chemoradiotherapy for Cervical Cancer Meta-Analysis, 2010)
- **Highlight:** Meta-analysis of chemoRT in cervical cancer
- **Design:**
  - Meta-analysis of randomized trials: RT (with or without surgery) vs. concomitant chemoRT (with or without surgery)
- **Results:**
  - On the basis of 13 RCTs that compared chemoRT vs. the same RT
    - 5% improvement in 5-yr survival with chemoRT (p < 0.001)
    - Larger survival benefit for two further trials, in which CT administered after chemoRT (Kantaradzic et al., 2004; Peters et al., 2000)
    - Significant survival benefit for trials that used platinum-based (HR = 0.83; p = 0.017) and non-platinum-based (HR = 0.77; p = 0.009) chemoRT
    - But no e/o difference in size of benefit by dosing or scheduling
    - ChemoRT reduced local and distant recurrences and progression
    - Acute hematological and GI toxicity increased with chemoRT; data too sparse for analysis of late toxicity
- **Conclusion:**
  - → Cochrane meta-analysis endorses chemoRT; even benefit of non-platinum-based CT; e/o benefit of adjuvant CT requires further testing in RCTs

Study: Ryu study

- **Citation:** (Ryu et al., 2011)
- **Highlight:** Weekly vs. q 3 wks cisplatin
- **Design:**
  - In phase II trial, 104 patients with stage IIB–IVA cervical cancer randomized to cisplatin 40 mg/m^2 q wk × 6 C vs. cisplatin 75 mg/m^2 q 3 wks × 3 C during concurrent RT (EBRT and ICBT)
- **Results:**
  - Compliance with treatment: 86.3% vs. 92.5% (p > 0.05) (weekly vs. tri-weekly)
  - Grade 3–4 neutropenia: 39.2% vs. 22.6% (p = 0.03)
  - 5-yr PFS: 70.6% vs. 75.5%
    - Mostly distal recurrences: 13/15 vs. 9/13
  - 5-yr OS: 66.5% vs. 88.7% (p = 0.03)
- **Conclusion:**
  - → Tri-weekly cisplatin 75 mg/m^2 CT concurrent with RT more effective and feasible than conventional weekly cisplatin 40 mg/m^2 in locally advanced cervical cancer

Study: Duenas-Gonzalez trial

- **Citation:** (Duenas-Gonzalez et al., 2003)
- **Highlight:** NACT carbo/Taxol, then radical hysterectomy and adjuvant cisRT
- **Design:**
  - Phase II: 43 patients with stage IB2–IIIB cervical cancer received carboplatin AUC 6 and paclitaxel 175 mg/m^2 over 3 hrs q 3 wks × 3 C, then underwent radical hysterectomy and adjuvant CTRT with cisplatin 40 mg/m^2 q wk × 6 C and concurrent EBRT, mean dose 49.3 Gy, and BCT with 32 Gy
- **Results:**
  - Toxicity NACT
    - Grade 3 and 4 neutropenia: 12% and 3%
    - Overall well-tolerated
  - Toxicity adjuvant CTRT
    - Mainly hematological and GI, mostly grade 1 and 2
  - 39/43 completed scheduled treatment
  - Evaluated for response to neoadjuvant CT
  - Response, clinically: 86% PR; 9% CR
  - 41/43 underwent radical hysterectomy
  - Response, pathologically: CR 17%, near CR 20%, 12% with positive surgical margins, and 20% with positive PLND
  - 26 patients scheduled for adjuvant CTRT
- **Conclusion:**
  - → Triple modality of NACT followed by radical hysterectomy and adjuvant CTRT is highly active treatment for locally advanced cervical cancer with acceptable toxicity

Study: Duenas-Gonzalez study II

- **Citation:** (Duenas-Gonzalez et al., 2011)
- **Highlight:** Locally advanced cervical cancer, CTRT, and adjuvant CT with cisplatin/gemcitabine
- **Design:**
  - 515 patients with stage IIB to IVA cervical cancer randomized to arm A (cisplatin 40 mg/m^2 and gemcitabine 125 mg/m^2 q wk × 6 wks with concurrent EBRT of 50.4 Gy in 28 fractions followed by BCT of 30–35 Gy in 96 hrs, and then 2 C of adjuvant cisplatin on day 1 and gemcitabine 1,000 mg/m^2 on days 1 and 8 q 3 wks) vs. arm B (cisplatin and concurrent EBRT followed by BCT; same dosing of concurrent CT as in arm A)
- **Results:**
  - Toxicities more frequent in arm A
    - Grade 3 and 4 toxicities: 86.5% vs. 46.3%; including two deaths possibly related to treatment toxicity in arm A

- – Predominantly hematologic side effects (neutropenia)
- – More discontinuations in arm A (p < 0.001)
- – In arm A, 86.2% received at least one cycle of adjuvant CT and 76.5% received both cycles
- – Late complications generally low
- • 3-yr PFS: 74.4% vs. 65% (p = 0.029)
- • Improved time to PD (p = 0.001)
- • Improved OS (HR = 0.68; p = 0.022)
- **Conclusion:**
  - • → Gemcitabine plus cisplatin chemoRT followed by BCT and adjuvant gemcitabine/cisplatin CT improved survival with increased but manageable toxicity

Study: INTERTECC-2

- • **Citation:** (Mell et al., 2017)
- • **Highlight:** Bone marrow-sparing IMRT
- • **Design:**
  - • Phase II trial: 83 patients with stage IB–IVA cervical cancer received cisplatin q wk and concurrent once-daily IMRT (followed by ICBT as indicated)
  - • Preplanned subgroup to test hypothesis that positron emission tomography-based image-guided IMRT (IG-IMRT) lowers risk of acute neutropenia
- • **Results:**
  - • Median follow-up: 26 months
  - • Incidence of any event: 26.5% compared to 40% incidence hypothesized from historical data (p = 0.012)
  - • Incidence of ≥ grade 3 neutropenia: 19.3%; clinically significant GI toxicity 12%
  - • With IG-IMRT (n = 35) vs. without IG-IMRT (n = 48)
    - – ≥ Grade 3 neutropenia: 8.6% vs. 27.1% (p = 0.035)
    - – ≥ Grade 3 leukopenia: 25.7% vs. 41.7% (p = 0.13)
    - – Any ≥ grade 3 hematologic toxicity: 31.4% vs. 43.8% (p = 0.25)
- • **Conclusion:**
  - • → IMRT reduces acute hematologic and GI toxicity compared with standard treatment; IG-IMRT reduces incidence of acute neutropenia

Study: Shrivastava trial

- • **Citation:** (Shrivastava et al., 2018)
- • **Highlight:** ChemoRT vs. RT in stage IIIB
- • **Design:**
  - • 850 patients with stage IIIB cervical cancer randomized to RT comprising EBRT (50 Gy in 25 fractions over 5 wks) and ICBT vs. same RT plus concurrent cisplatin 40 mg/m² q wk for at least × 5 C

- **Results:**
  - Median follow-up: 88 months
  - 69.1% received at least 5 C of cisplatin
  - Higher incidence of hematologic AE in CTRT arm
  - 5-yr DFS: 52.3% vs. 43.8% (p = 0.03) (CTRT vs. RT)
  - 5-yr OS: 54% vs. 46% (p = 0.04)
  - After adjusting for prognostic factors, CTRT continued to be significantly superior to RT in DFS and OS
- **Conclusion:**
  - → CTRT using weekly cisplatin resulted in better DFS and OS compared to RT in stage IIIB cervical cancer (largest clinical trial so far in favor of concurrent weekly cisRT)

Study: GOG 263/KGOG 1008

- **Citation:** Ongoing (NCT01101451)
- **Design:**
  - Patients with stage IA, IB, and IIA cervical cancer s/p radical hysterectomy and PLND with intermediate-risk factors randomized to pelvic EBRT or IMRT qd 5 d a week for 5.5 wks plus weekly cisplatin 40 mg/m^2 for up to 6 C vs. EBRT or IMRT alone (same regimen)
  - Definition of intermediate risk and thus eligibility = GOG 92

Study: TACO trial/KGOG 1027

- **Citation:** Ongoing (NCT01561586)
- **Background:**
  - Tri-weekly cisplatin-based chemoradiation in locally advanced cervical cancer
- **Design:**
  - Patients with stages IB2 and IIB–IVA cervical cancer randomized to cisplatin 40 mg/m^2 q wk × 6 plus concurrent RT vs. cisplatin 75 mg/m^2 q 3 wks × 3 C plus concurrent RT

3.4 STUDIES ADDRESSING TREATMENT OF RECURRENT OR METASTATIC CERVICAL CANCER

3.4.1 Chemotherapy and Targeted Therapy

Study: GOG 169

- **Citation:** (Moore et al., 2004)
- **Highlight:** Cisplatin (C) vs. cisplatin + paclitaxel (C + P)

- **Design:**
  - 264 patients with stage IVB, recurrent, or persistent squamous cell carcinoma of cervix randomized to cisplatin 50 mg/m² q 3 wks × 6 C vs. cisplatin 50 mg/m² plus paclitaxel 135 mg/m² q 3 wks × 6 C
- **Results:**
  - Majority had prior RT (C 92% vs. C + P 91%)
  - Grade 3 and 4 anemia and neutropenia more common in combination arm
  - No significant difference in QoL scores, although disproportionate number dropped out in both arms
  - ORR: 19% (6% CR; 13% PR) vs. 36% (15% CR; 21% PR) (p = 0.002)
  - Median PFS: 2.8 vs. 4.8 months (p < 0.001)
  - No difference in median OS: 8.8 vs. 9.7 months
- **Conclusion:**
  - → C + P superior to cisplatin alone in response rate and PFS with sustained QoL

Study: GOG 179

- **Citation:** (Long et al., 2005)
- **Highlight:** Cisplatin vs. cisplatin + topotecan
- **Design:**
  - 294 patients with stage IVB, recurrent, or persistent cervical cancer randomized to cisplatin 50 mg/m² q 3 wks (CPT) vs. cisplatin 50 mg/m² day 1 plus topotecan 0.75 mg/m² days 1 and 3 q 3 wks (CT) vs. methotrexate (MTX) 30 mg/m² days 1, 15, and 22, vinblastine 3 mg/m² days 2, 15, and 22, doxorubicin 30 mg/m² day 2, and cisplatin 70 mg/m² day 2 q 4 wks (MVAC)
- **Results:**
  - MVAC arm was closed after four treatment-related deaths (4/63)
  - 146 patients received CPT; 147 CT
  - Grade 3 and 4 hematologic toxicities more common in CT
  - Response rates: 13% vs. 27% (CPT vs. CT)
  - Median PFS: 2.9 vs. 4.6 months (p = 0.014)
  - Median OS: 6.5 vs. 9.4 months (p = 0.017)
- **Conclusion:**
  - → First randomized phase III trial demonstrating survival advantage for combination CT over cisplatin alone in advanced cervical cancer

Study: GOG 204

- **Citation:** (Monk et al., 2009)
- **Highlight:** Paclitaxel (PC) vs. vinorelbine (VC) vs. gemcitabine (GC) vs. topotecan (TC)
- **Design:**
  - 513 patients with advanced and recurrent cervical cancer randomized to four cisplatin-containing doublet combinations

- – PC: Paclitaxel 135 mg/m^2 over 24 hrs plus cisplatin 50 mg/m^2 on day 2 q 3 wks
- – VC: Vinorelbine 30 mg/m^2 days 1 and 8 plus cisplatin 50 mg/m^2 on day 1 q 3 wks
- – GC: Gemcitabine 1,000 mg/m^2 days 1 and 8 plus cisplatin 50 mg/m^2 on day 1 q 3 wks
- – TC: Topotecan 0.75 mg/m^2 days 1, 2, and 3 plus cisplatin 50 mg/m^2 on day 1 q 3 wks
- **Results:**
  - Response rates: 29.1%, 25.9%, 22.3%, and 23.4% for PC, VC, GC, TC
  - Experimental-to-PC HR for PFS: 1.36 (CI: 0.97–1.9) for VC, 1.39 (CI: 0.99–1.96) for GC, and 1.27 (CI: 0.9–1.78) for TC
  - Experimental-to-PC HR for death: 1.15 (CI: 0.79–1.69) for VC, 1.32 (CI: 0.91–1.92) for GC, and 1.26 (CI: 0.86–1.82) for TC
  - All arms comparable in toxicity except
    - – Fewer grade 3 or 4 leukopenia in GC arm
    - – More grade 2 alopecia in PC (54%; p < 0.0001)
- **Conclusion:**
  - → VC, GC, and TC not superior to PC in OS; trend in RR, PFS, and OS favors PC

Study: GOG 240

- **Citation:** (Tewari et al., 2014)
- **Highlight:** Addition of BEV
- **Design:**
  - 452 patients with recurrent, persistent, or metastatic cervical cancer randomized to two groups of CT alone and two groups of CT plus BEV
    - – Cisplatin: 50 mg/m^2 plus paclitaxel 135 or 175 mg/m^2 (CP)
    - – Topotecan: 0.75 mg/m^2 days 1–3 plus paclitaxel 175 mg/m^2 (TP)
    - – Cisplatin: 50 mg/m^2 plus paclitaxel 135 or 175 mg/m^2 plus BEV 15 mg/kg
    - – Topotecan: 0.75 mg/m^2 days 1–3 plus paclitaxel 175 mg/m^2 plus BEV 15 mg/kg
- **Results:**
  - BEV associated with increased incidence
    - – ≥ Grade 2 hypertension: 25% vs. 2%
    - – ≥ Grade 3 thromboembolic events: 8% vs. 1%
    - – ≥ Grade 3 GI fistulas: 3% vs. 0%
  - At interim analysis with median follow-up of 12.5 months
    - – Higher risk of progression for TP compared to CP (HR = 1.39 [CI: 1.09–1.77])
    - – But no difference in OS (HR for death 1.2 [CI: 0.82–1.76]); also, no difference in mortality between the CT regimens with previous exposure to platinum

- – With previous exposure: HR = 1.18 (CI: 0.84–1.65)
  - – Without previous exposure: HR = 1.35 (CI: 0.68–2.69)
- Data for the two CT regimens combined analyzing addition of BEV
  - – Median follow-up: 20.8 months
  - – Median OS: 17.0 vs. 13.3 months (HR for death 0.71 [CI = 0.54–0.95]; p = 0.004) (CT + BEV vs. CT alone)
  - – Median PFS: 8.2 vs. 5.9 months (HR = 0.67 [CI = 0.54–0.82])
  - – Response rate: 48% vs. 36% (p = 0.008); + BEV: CR in 28 patients; – BEV: CR in 14 patients (p = 0.03)
    - – CP + BEV compared to CP alone: HR for death 0.68 (CI = 0.48–0.97) and response rates: 50% vs. 45% (p = 0.51)
    - – TP + BEV compared to TP alone: HR for death 0.74 (CI = 0.53–1.05) and response rates: 47% vs. 27% (p = 0.002)
- **Conclusion:**
  - → Addition of BEV to combination CT in recurrent, persistent, and metastatic cervical cancer associated with improved OS by 3.7 months

Study: GOG 240

- **Citation:** (Tewari et al., 2017)
- **Highlight:** Addition of BEV long-term results
- **Results:**
  - Median OS: 16.8 vs. 13.3 months (HR 0.77 [CI = 0.62–0.95]; p = 0.0068 (+ BEV vs. – BEV)
    - – OS among patients not treated with prior pelvic RT: 24.5 vs. 16.8 months
  - Median PFS: HR 0.68 (CI = 0.56–0.84); p = 0.0002
  - Median post-progression OS: 8.4 vs. 7.1 months (HR 0.32 [CI = 0.66–1.05]; p = 0.06)
  - Fistulas of any grade in 14.5% (all radiated previously)
    - – ≥ Grade 3 fistulas in 5.9% and did not result in surgical emergency
- **Conclusion:**
  - → Benefit of BEV sustained with extended follow-up; no negative rebound after progression

Study: JGOG 0505

- **Citation:** (Kitagawa et al., 2015)
- **Highlight:** Cisplatin + paclitaxel vs. carboplatin + paclitaxel
- **Design:**
  - 253 patients with metastatic or recurrent cervical cancer that had ≤1 platinum-containing treatment and no prior taxane randomized to conventional paclitaxel plus cisplatin (TP; paclitaxel 135 mg/m^2 over 24 hrs on day 1 and cisplatin 50 mg/m^2 on day 2 q 3 wks) vs. paclitaxel plus carboplatin (TC; paclitaxel 175 mg/m^2 over 3 hrs and carboplatin AUC 5 mg/mL/min on day 1 q 3 wks)

- **Results:**
  - HR for OS: 0.994 (CI: 0.79–1.25); non-inferiority (p = 0.032)
  - Median OS: 18.3 vs. 17.5 months (TP vs. TC)
    - Among patients without prior cisplatin: median OS: 23.2 vs. 13 months (HR 1.57 [CI = 1.06–2.32])
    - One treatment-related death in TC group
    - Proportion of non-hospitalization periods greater with TC (p < 0.001)
- **Conclusion:**
  - → Paclitaxel plus carboplatin non-inferior to paclitaxel plus cisplatin and should be standard treatment for metastatic or recurrent cervical cancer
  - However, cisplatin still key drug for patients who have not received platinum agents

Study: InnovaTV 204/GOG 3023/ENGOT-cx6

- **Citation:** (Coleman et al., 2021)
- **Highlight:** Tisotumab vedotin
- **Design:**
  - In open-label phase II trial, 101 patients with recurrent, metastatic, or progressive cervical cancer; ≤2 prior lines received 2.0 mg/kg (up to a maximum of 200 mg) tisotumab vedotin iv q 3 wks until progression or toxicity
  - Tisotumab vedotin: antibody drug conjugate binds to tissue factor (TF, or thromboplastin, or CD142) on target cells; TF highly prevalent on multiple solid tumors, including cervical cancer; upon internalization, tisotumab releases monomethyl auristatin E (MMAE), a microtubule-disrupting agent resulting in cell-cycle arrest and apoptosis
- **Results:**
  - Median follow-up: 10.0 months
  - ORR: 24% (7 CR; 17 PR)
  - Median DOR: 8.3 months
  - DCR: 72%
  - Median PFS: 4.2 months
  - Median OS: 12.1 months
  - ≥ Grade 3 AEs in 28%
    - Neutropenia: 3%
    - Fatigue: 2%
    - Ulcerative keratitis: 2%
    - Peripheral neuropathy: 13%
- **Conclusion:**
  - Tisotumab showed meaningful and durable antitumor activity with manageable safety profile

3.4.2 Immunotherapy

Study: Checkmate 358

- **Citation:** (Naumann et al., 2019a)
- **Highlight:** Nivolumab monotherapy in virus-associated tumors
- **Design:**
  - Multicohort phase I/II study of nivolumab 240 mg q 2 wks in patients with virus-associated tumors; here, results for recurrent or metastatic cervical, vaginal, and vulvar cancer, with ≤2 prior lines; PD-L1 unselected
- **Results:**
  - 19 patients with cervical cancer; five with vaginal or vulvar cancer
  - ORR: 26.3% for cervical cancer and 20% for vaginal/vulvar cancer
  - DCR: 68.4% for cervical cancer and 80% for vaginal/vulvar cancer
  - In cervical cancer, response regardless of PD-L1 or HPV status or number of prior lines
  - At median follow-up of 19.2 months, median DOR not reached in cervical cancer and 5 months in vaginal/vulvar cancer
  - Median PFS: 5.1 months in cervical cancer
  - Median OS: 21.9 months in cervical cancer
  - ≥ Grade 3 AEs: 21.1%
- **Conclusion:**
  - → Nivolumab with encouraging clinical activity and manageable safety profile

Study: Checkmate 358

- **Citation:** NCT02488759; ongoing; abstract presented at ESMO 2019 (Naumann et al., 2019b)
- **Highlight:** Nivo + ipi
- **Design:**
  - Multicohort phase I/II study of nivo +/– ipi in patients with virus-associated tumors regardless of PD-L1 expression
  - Here, interim analysis or recurrent or metastatic cervical with zero to two prior lines
  - Patients randomized to nivo 3 mg/kg q 2 wks + ipi 1 mg/kg q 6 wks (combo A) vs. nivo 1 mg/kg + ipi 3 mg/kg q 3 wks × 4 doses followed by nivo 240 mg q 2 wks (combo B), for ≤24 months until progression or toxicity
- **Results:**
  - Median follow-up: 13.9 and 10.7 months (combo B vs. A)
  - ORR
    - Without prior systemic treatment: 46% vs. 32%
    - With prior systemic treatment: 36% vs. 23%

- Median PFS
  - Without prior systemic treatment: 8.5 vs. 13.8 months
  - With prior systemic treatment: 5.8 vs. 3.6 months
- Median OS
  - Without prior systemic treatment: NR vs. NR
  - With prior systemic treatment: 25.4 vs. 10.3 months
- ≥ Grade 3 AE: 37% vs. 28.9%
- **Conclusion:**
  - → Clinical benefit from two regimens of nivo + ipi in recurrent/metastatic cervical cancer regardless of PD-L1 status; combo B with notable efficacy in patients with prior systemic treatment

Study: Keynote-158

- **Citation:** (Chung et al., 2019)
- **Highlight:** Pembrolizumab in advanced cervical cancer
- **Design:**
  - Phase II basket study on pembrolizumab 200 mg q 3 wks in 11 cancer types; here, interim results on 98 patients in the cervical cancer cohort with progression or intolerance to ≥1 line
  - PD-L1 positivity defined as combined positive score (CPS) ≥1
- **Results:**
  - 98 patients treated: 65.3% with ECOG 1
    - 93.9% with metastatic disease
    - 83.7% with PD-L1-positive tumors (CPS ≥1)
  - Median follow-up: 10.3 months
  - ORR: 12.2% (14.6% for PD-L1-positive tumors)
    - 3 CR
    - 9 PR (all 12 responses in PD-L1-positive tumors)
    - Median DOR not reached
    - 18 SD (15 in PD-L1-positive tumors)
  - DCR: 30.6%
  - Median PFS: 2.1 months
  - Median OS: 9.4 months
  - Most common AEs
    - Hypothyroidism: 10.2%
    - Decreased appetite: 9.2%
    - Fatigue: 9.2%
  - ≥ Grade 3 AEs: 12.2%
- **Conclusion:**
  - → Pembrolizumab monotherapy with durable antitumor activity and manageable safety

Study: Keynote-826

- **Citation:** (Colombo et al., 2021)
- **Highlight:** Pembrolizumab + CT

- **Design:**
  - 548 patients with persistent, recurrent, or metastatic cervical cancer randomized to pembrolizumab 200 mg q 3 wks for up to 35 cycles plus platinum-based CT (limited to six cycles in second protocol amendment) ± BEV vs. placebo plus platinum-based CT ± BEV
  - Interim analysis
- **Results:**
  - Median PFS
    - In 548 patients with CPS ≥1: 10.4 vs. 8.2 months (HR 0.62 [CI = 0.5–0.77]; p < 0.001)
    - In 617 patients in intention-to-treat population: 10.4 vs. 8.2 months (HR 0.65 [CI = 0.53–0.79]; p < 0.001)
    - In 317 patients with CPS ≥10: 10.4 vs. 8.1 months (HR 0.58 [CI = 0.44–0.77]; p < 0.001)
  - 2-yrs OS
    - In 548 patients with CPS ≥1: 53% vs. 41.7% (HR 0.64 [CI = 0.5–0.81]; p < 0.001)
    - In 617 patients in intention-to-treat population: 50.4% vs. 40.4% (HR 0.67 [CI = 0.54–0.84]; p < 0.001)
    - In 317 patients with CPS ≥10: 54.4% vs. 44.6% (HR 0.61 [CI = 0.44–0.84]; p < 0.001)
  - Most common ≥ grade 3 AE
    - Anemia: 30.3% vs. 26.9% (pembrolizumab vs. placebo)
    - Neutropenia: 12.4% vs. 9.7%
- **Conclusion:**
  - → PFS and OS significantly longer with pembrolizumab

Study: GOG 3016/ENGOT En-Cx9

- **Citation:** (Tewari et al., 2022)
- **Highlight:** Cemiplimab
- **Design:**
  - 608 patients with recurrent cervical cancer regardless of PD-L1 status randomized to 350 mg cemiplimab q 3 wks vs. investigator-choice single-agent CT
  - Cemiplimab: PD-1 antibody
- **Results:**
  - ORR: 16.4% vs. 6.3%
    - ORR: 18% in PD-L1 ≥1% and 11% in PD-L1 <1%
  - Median PFS: 2.8 vs. 2.9 months (HR 0.75 [CI = 0.63–0.89]; p < 0.001)
  - Median OS: 12.0 vs. 8.5 months (HR 0.69 [CI = 0.56–0.84]; p < 0.001)
    - OS benefit consistent in both histological subgroups (squamous and adenoca)
  - ≥ Grade 3 AEs: 45% vs. 53.4%
- **Conclusion:**
  - → Survival was significantly longer with cemiplimab than with single-agent CT in recurrent cervical cancer after first-line platinum-containing CT

Study: Study C-145-04

- **Citation:** NCT03108495; ongoing; presented at ASCO 2019 (Jazaeri et al., 2019)
- **Highlight:** TILs (LN-145)
- **Design:**
  - In open-label phase 2 trial, patients with recurrent, metastatic, or persistent cervical cancer and ≥1 prior line receive adoptive cell transfer using tumor-infiltrating lymphocytes (TILs)
  - Tumor surgically harvested and shipped to central facility for TIL generation; 22-day manufacturing process; final TIL product cryopreserved and shipped; 1 wk of preconditioning lymphodepletion with cyclophosphamide and fludarabine; single LN-145 infusion, followed by up to six doses of 600,000 IU/kg IL-2
- **Results:**
  - ORR: 44% (1 CR; 9 PR; 2 unconfirmed PR)
  - DCR: 89% at median follow-up of 3.5 months
- **Conclusion:**
  - → LN-145 offers viable therapeutic option in recurrent, metastatic cervical cancer

REFERENCES

Chemoradiotherapy for Cervical Cancer Meta-Analysis, C. (2010). Reducing uncertainties about the effects of chemoradiotherapy for cervical cancer: individual patient data meta-analysis. Cochrane Database Syst Rev, CD008285. 10.1002/14651858.CD008285.

Chung, H.C., Ros, W., Delord, J.P., Perets, R., Italiano, A., Shapira-Frommer, R., Manzuk, L., Piha-Paul, S.A., Xu, L., Zeigenfuss, S., et al. (2019). Efficacy and safety of pembrolizumab in previously treated advanced cervical cancer: results from the phase II KEYNOTE-158 study. J Clin Oncol 37, 1470–1478. 10.1200/JCO.18.01265.

Coleman, R.L., Lorusso, D., Gennigens, C., Gonzalez-Martin, A., Randall, L., Cibula, D., Lund, B., Woelber, L., Pignata, S., Forget, F., et al. (2021). Efficacy and safety of tisotumab vedotin in previously treated recurrent or metastatic cervical cancer (innovaTV 204/GOG-3023/ENGOT-cx6): a multicentre, open-label, single-arm, phase 2 study. Lancet Oncol 22, 609–619. 10.1016/S1470-2045(21)00056-5.

Colombo, N., Dubot, C., Lorusso, D., Caceres, M.V., Hasegawa, K., Shapira-Frommer, R., Tewari, K.S., Salman, P., Hoyos Usta, E., Yanez, E., et al. (2021). Pembrolizumab for persistent, recurrent, or metastatic cervical cancer. N Engl J Med 385, 1856–1867. 10.1056/NEJMoa2112435.

Delgado, G., Bundy, B.N., Fowler, W.C., Jr., Stehman, F.B., Sevin, B., Creasman, W.T., Major, F., DiSaia, P., and Zaino, R. (1989). A prospective surgical pathological study of stage I squamous carcinoma of the cervix: a Gynecologic Oncology Group study. Gynecol Oncol 35, 314–320.

Delgado, G., Bundy, B., Zaino, R., Sevin, B.U., Creasman, W.T., and Major, F. (1990). Prospective surgical-pathological study of disease-free interval in patients with stage IB squamous cell carcinoma of the cervix: a Gynecologic Oncology Group study. Gynecol Oncol 38, 352–357.

Duenas-Gonzalez, A., Lopez-Graniel, C., Gonzalez-Enciso, A., Cetina, L., Rivera, L., Mariscal, I., Montalvo, G., Gomez, E., de la Garza, J., Chanona, G., and Mohar, A. (2003). A phase II study of multimodality treatment for locally advanced cervical cancer: neoadjuvant carboplatin and paclitaxel followed by radical hysterectomy and adjuvant cisplatin chemoradiation. Ann Oncol *14*, 1278–1284.

Duenas-Gonzalez, A., Zarba, J.J., Patel, F., Alcedo, J.C., Beslija, S., Casanova, L., Pattaranutaporn, P., Hameed, S., Blair, J.M., Barraclough, H., and Orlando, M. (2011). Phase III, open-label, randomized study comparing concurrent gemcitabine plus cisplatin and radiation followed by adjuvant gemcitabine and cisplatin versus concurrent cisplatin and radiation in patients with stage IIB to IVA carcinoma of the cervix. J Clin Oncol *29*, 1678–1685. 10.1200/JCO.2009.25.9663.

Eifel, P.J., Winter, K., Morris, M., Levenback, C., Grigsby, P.W., Cooper, J., Rotman, M., Gershenson, D., and Mutch, D.G. (2004). Pelvic irradiation with concurrent chemotherapy versus pelvic and para-aortic irradiation for high-risk cervical cancer: an update of Radiation Therapy Oncology Group trial (RTOG) 90–01. J Clin Oncol *22*, 872–880. 10.1200/JCO.2004.07.197.

Frumovitz, M., Obermair, A., Coleman, R.L., Pareja, R., Lopez, A., Ribero, R., Isla, D., Rendon, G., Bernardini, M.Q., Buda, A., et al. (2020). Quality of life in patients with cervical cancer after open versus minimally invasive radical hysterectomy (LACC): a secondary outcome of a multicentre, randomised, open-label, phase 3, non-inferiority trial. Lancet Oncol *21*, 851–860. 10.1016/S1470-2045(20)30081-4.

Jazaeri, A.A., Zsiros, E., Amaria, R.N., Artz, A.S., Edwards, R.P., Wenham, R.M., Slomovitz, B.M., Walther, A., Thomas, S.S., Chesney, J.A., et al. (2019). Safety and efficacy of adoptive cell transfer using autologous tumor infiltrating lymphocytes (LN-145) for treatment of recurrent, metastatic, or persistent cervical carcinoma. J Clin Oncol *37*, 2538–2538. 10.1200/JCO.2019.37.15_suppl.2538.

Kantaradzic, N., Beslija, S., and Kalamujic, M. (2004). Comparison of gastrointestinal toxicity in patients with advanced cervical carcinoma treated with concomitant chemotherapy and radiotherapy versus radiotherapy alone. Med Arh *58*, 214–217.

Keys, H.M., Bundy, B.N., Stehman, F.B., Muderspach, L.I., Chafe, W.E., Suggs, C.L., 3rd, Walker, J.L., and Gersell, D. (1999). Cisplatin, radiation, and adjuvant hysterectomy compared with radiation and adjuvant hysterectomy for bulky stage IB cervical carcinoma. N Engl J Med *340*, 1154–1161. 10.1056/NEJM199904153401503.

Keys, H.M., Bundy, B.N., Stehman, F.B., Okagaki, T., Gallup, D.G., Burnett, A.F., Rotman, M.Z., Fowler, W.C., Jr., and Gynecologic Oncology Group. (2003). Radiation therapy with and without extrafascial hysterectomy for bulky stage IB cervical carcinoma: a randomized trial of the Gynecologic Oncology Group. Gynecol Oncol *89*, 343–353.

Kitagawa, R., Katsumata, N., Shibata, T., Kamura, T., Kasamatsu, T., Nakanishi, T., Nishimura, S., Ushijima, K., Takano, M., Satoh, T., and Yoshikawa, H. (2015). Paclitaxel plus carboplatin versus paclitaxel plus cisplatin in metastatic or recurrent cervical cancer: the open-label randomized phase III trial JCOG0505. J Clin Oncol *33*, 2129–2135. 10.1200/JCO.2014.58.4391.

Landoni, F., Maneo, A., Colombo, A., Placa, F., Milani, R., Perego, P., Favini, G., Ferri, L., and Mangioni, C. (1997). Randomised study of radical surgery versus radiotherapy for stage Ib-IIa cervical cancer. Lancet *350*, 535–540. 10.1016/S0140-6736(97)02250-2.

Long, H.J., 3rd, Bundy, B.N., Grendys, E.C., Jr., Benda, J.A., McMeekin, D.S., Sorosky, J., Miller, D.S., Eaton, L.A., Fiorica, J.V., and Gynecologic Oncology Group, S. (2005). Randomized phase III trial of cisplatin with or without topotecan in carcinoma of the uterine cervix: a Gynecologic Oncology Group study. J Clin Oncol *23*, 4626–4633. 10.1200/JCO.2005.10.021.

Mell, L.K., Sirak, I., Wei, L., Tarnawski, R., Mahantshetty, U., Yashar, C.M., McHale, M.T., Xu, R., Honerkamp-Smith, G., Carmona, R., et al. (2017). Bone marrow-sparing intensity modulated radiation therapy with concurrent cisplatin for stage IB-IVA cervical cancer: an international multicenter phase II clinical trial (INTERTECC-2). Int J Radiat Oncol Biol Phys *97*, 536–545. 10.1016/j.ijrobp.2016.11.027.

Mileshkin, L.R., Moore, K.N., Barnes, E., Gebski, V., Narayan, K., Bradshaw, N., Lee, Y.C., Diamante, K., Fyles, A.W., Small, W., et al. (2021). Adjuvant chemotherapy following chemoradiation as primary treatment for locally advanced cervical cancer compared to chemoradiation alone: the randomized phase III OUTBACK trial (ANZGOG 0902, RTOG 1174, NRG 0274). J Clin Oncol 39, LBA3–LBA3. 10.1200/JCO.2021.39.15_suppl.LBA3.

Monk, B.J., Sill, M.W., McMeekin, D.S., Cohn, D.E., Ramondetta, L.M., Boardman, C.H., Benda, J., and Cella, D. (2009). Phase III trial of four cisplatin-containing doublet combinations in stage IVB, recurrent, or persistent cervical carcinoma: a Gynecologic Oncology Group study. J Clin Oncol 27, 4649–4655. 10.1200/JCO.2009.21.8909.

Moore, D.H., Blessing, J.A., McQuellon, R.P., Thaler, H.T., Cella, D., Benda, J., Miller, D.S., Olt, G., King, S., Boggess, J.F., and Rocereto, T.F. (2004). Phase III study of cisplatin with or without paclitaxel in stage IVB, recurrent, or persistent squamous cell carcinoma of the cervix: a Gynecologic Oncology Group study. J Clin Oncol 22, 3113–3119. 10.1200/JCO.2004.04.170.

Morris, M., Eifel, P.J., Lu, J., Grigsby, P.W., Levenback, C., Stevens, R.E., Rotman, M., Gershenson, D.M., and Mutch, D.G. (1999). Pelvic radiation with concurrent chemotherapy compared with pelvic and para-aortic radiation for high-risk cervical cancer. N Engl J Med 340, 1137–1143. 10.1056/NEJM199904153401501.

Naumann, R.W., Hollebecque, A., Meyer, T., Devlin, M.J., Oaknin, A., Kerger, J., Lopez-Picazo, J.M., Machiels, J.P., Delord, J.P., Evans, T.R.J., et al. (2019a). Safety and efficacy of nivolumab monotherapy in recurrent or metastatic cervical, vaginal, or vulvar carcinoma: results from the phase I/II checkmate 358 trial. J Clin Oncol 37, 2825–2834. 10.1200/JCO.19.00739.

Naumann, R.W., Oaknin, A., Meyer, T., Lopez-Picazo, J.M., Lao, C., Bang, Y., Boni, V., Sharfman, W.H., Park, J.C., Devriese, L., Harano, K., Chung, C.H., Topalian, S.L., Zaki, K., Chen, T., Gu, J., Li, B., Barrows, A.M., Horvath, A., Moore, K.N. (2019b). Efficacy and safety of nivolumab (Nivo) + ipilimumab (Ipi) in patients (pts) with recurrent/metastatic (R/M) cervical cancer: results from CheckMate 358. ESMO. Ann Oncol 30 (suppl_5), v851–v934. 10.1093/annonc/mdz394.

Peters, W.A., 3rd, Liu, P.Y., Barrett, R.J., 2nd, Stock, R.J., Monk, B.J., Berek, J.S., Souhami, L., Grigsby, P., Gordon, W., Jr., and Alberts, D.S. (2000). Concurrent chemotherapy and pelvic radiation therapy compared with pelvic radiation therapy alone as adjuvant therapy after radical surgery in high-risk early-stage cancer of the cervix. J Clin Oncol 18, 1606–1613. 10.1200/JCO.2000.18.8.1606.

Ramirez, P.T., Frumovitz, M., Pareja, R., Lopez, A., Vieira, M., Ribeiro, R., Buda, A., Yan, X., Shuzhong, Y., Chetty, N., et al. (2018). Minimally invasive versus abdominal radical hysterectomy for cervical cancer. N Engl J Med 379, 1895–1904. 10.1056/NEJMoa1806395.

Rose, P.G., Bundy, B.N., Watkins, E.B., Thigpen, J.T., Deppe, G., Maiman, M.A., Clarke-Pearson, D.L., and Insalaco, S. (1999). Concurrent cisplatin-based radiotherapy and chemotherapy for locally advanced cervical cancer. N Engl J Med 340, 1144–1153. 10.1056/NEJM199904153401502.

Rotman, M., Choi, K., Guse, C., Marcial, V., Hornback, N., and John, M. (1990). Prophylactic irradiation of the para-aortic lymph node chain in stage IIB and bulky stage IB carcinoma of the cervix, initial treatment results of RTOG 7920. Int J Radiat Oncol Biol Phys 19, 513–521.

Rotman, M., Pajak, T.F., Choi, K., Clery, M., Marcial, V., Grigsby, P.W., Cooper, J., and John, M. (1995). Prophylactic extended-field irradiation of para-aortic lymph nodes in stages IIB and bulky IB and IIA cervical carcinomas. Ten-year treatment results of RTOG 79–20. JAMA 274, 387–393.

Rotman, M., Sedlis, A., Piedmonte, M.R., Bundy, B., Lentz, S.S., Muderspach, L.I., and Zaino, R.J. (2006). A phase III randomized trial of postoperative pelvic irradiation in Stage IB cervical carcinoma with poor prognostic features: follow-up of a Gynecologic Oncology Group study. Int J Radiat Oncol Biol Phys 65, 169–176. 10.1016/j.ijrobp.2005.10.019.

Ryu, S.Y., Lee, W.M., Kim, K., Park, S.I., Kim, B.J., Kim, M.H., Choi, S.C., Cho, C.K., Nam, B.H., and Lee, E.D. (2011). Randomized clinical trial of weekly vs. triweekly cisplatin-based chemotherapy concurrent with radiotherapy in the treatment of locally advanced cervical cancer. Int J Radiat Oncol Biol Phys *81*, e577–581. 10.1016/j.ijrobp.2011.05.002.

Sedlis, A., Bundy, B.N., Rotman, M.Z., Lentz, S.S., Muderspach, L.I., and Zaino, R.J. (1999). A randomized trial of pelvic radiation therapy versus no further therapy in selected patients with stage IB carcinoma of the cervix after radical hysterectomy and pelvic lymphade-nectomy: a Gynecologic Oncology Group study. Gynecol Oncol *73*, 177–183. 10.1006/gyno.1999.5387.

Shrivastava, S., Mahantshetty, U., Engineer, R., Chopra, S., Hawaldar, R., Hande, V., Kerkar, R.A., Maheshwari, A., Shylasree, T.S., Ghosh, J., et al. (2018, April 1). Cisplatin chemoradio-therapy vs radiotherapy in FIGO stage IIIB squamous cell carcinoma of the uterine cervix: a randomized clinical trial. JAMA Oncol *4* (4), 506–513. 10.1001/jamaoncol.2017.5179.

Stehman, F.B., Ali, S., Keys, H.M., Muderspach, L.I., Chafe, W.E., Gallup, D.G., Walker, J.L., and Gersell, D. (2007). Radiation therapy with or without weekly cisplatin for bulky stage 1B cervical carcinoma: follow-up of a Gynecologic Oncology Group trial. Am J Obstet Gynecol *197*, 503 e501–506. 10.1016/j.ajog.2007.08.003.

Tewari, K.S., Monk, B.J., Vergote, I., Miller, A., de Melo, A.C., Kim, H.S., Kim, Y.M., Lisyanskaya, A., Samouelian, V., Lorusso, D., et al. (2022). Survival with cemiplimab in recurrent cervical cancer. N Engl J Med *386*, 544–555. 10.1056/NEJMoa2112187.

Tewari, K.S., Sill, M.W., Long, H.J., 3rd, Penson, R.T., Huang, H., Ramondetta, L.M., Landrum, L.M., Oaknin, A., Reid, T.J., Leitao, M.M., et al. (2014). Improved survival with bevaci-zumab in advanced cervical cancer. N Engl J Med *370*, 734–743. 10.1056/NEJMoa1309748.

Tewari, K.S., Sill, M.W., Penson, R.T., Huang, H., Ramondetta, L.M., Landrum, L.M., Oaknin, A., Reid, T.J., Leitao, M.M., Michael, H.E., et al. (2017). Bevacizumab for advanced cervical cancer: final overall survival and adverse event analysis of a randomised, controlled, open-label, phase 3 trial (Gynecologic Oncology Group 240). Lancet *390*, 1654–1663. 10.1016/S0140–6736(17)31607-0.

Whitney, C.W., Sause, W., Bundy, B.N., Malfetano, J.H., Hannigan, E.V., Fowler, W.C., Jr., Clarke-Pearson, D.L., and Liao, S.Y. (1999). Randomized comparison of fluorouracil plus cisplatin versus hydroxyurea as an adjunct to radiation therapy in stage IIB-IVA carcinoma of the cervix with negative para-aortic lymph nodes: a Gynecologic Oncology Group and Southwest Oncology Group study. J Clin Oncol *17*, 1339–1348. 10.1200/JCO.1999.17.5.1339.

Vulvar Cancer

4

4.1 STUDIES ADDRESSING SURGICAL TREATMENT

Study: GOG 36

- **Citation:** (Sedlis et al., 1987)
- **Highlight:** Predictors of groin LN metastases in *superficial* vulvar cancer
- **Design:**
  - Interest in less radical treatment for low-risk vulvar cancer; however, unfavorable outcomes reported in patients with micro-invasive vulvar cancer; therefore, goal to investigate risk factors to define low-risk vulvar cancer suitable for conservative therapy
  - From 1977 to 1984, 558 patients with primary vulvar squamous cell carcinoma prospectively enrolled in GOG protocol 'Clinical Pathological Study of Vulvar Carcinoma' and treated by radical vulvectomy and bilateral groin node dissection
- **Results:**
  - 272/558 patients with superficial (≤5 mm) squamous cell vulvar carcinoma
    - 57/272 (21%) with positive groin LNs
    - 28/272 (10.3%) with ≥2 positive LNs
  - Analyzed: Tumor thickness, clinical tumor size, pathologic tumor size, tumor location, clinical node status, grade by author's criteria, conventional grade, capillary-like space involvement, and exophytic tumor growth
  - Linear logistic model showed significant predictors of groin LN metastasis:
    - Tumor thickness
      - Tumor thickness: From surface to deepest tumor penetration
    - Grade (as per author's criteria = GOG grading, according to the proportion of undifferentiated tumor)
      - G1: No poorly differentiated component; G2: ratio ≤1:3; G3: ratio >1:3 to ≤1:2; G4: ratio >1:2
    - Capillary-like space involvement
    - Clitoral and perineal location
    - Clinically suspicious LN

DOI: 10.1201/9781003229711-4

- Identified risk factors not entirely reliable when used alone but useful when combined in a formula (statistical model)
- Lowest risk for LN metastases (0 observed; 2% expected) in subset of patients with no clinically suspicious nodes, negative capillary-like space, non-midline vulvar cancer, either grade 1 and 1–5 mm thick or grade 2 and 1–2 mm thick (only about 25% of the examined patients in this group)
- **Conclusion:**
  - → Risk of LN metastases best determined by simultaneous evaluation of all risk factors rather than a single factor, such as tumor thickness

Study: GOG 36

- **Citation:** (Homesley et al., 1993)
- **Highlight:** Predictors of groin LN metastases in vulvar cancer *overall*
- **Design:**
  - Primary aim: To determine the validity of 1970 FIGO staging relative to various clinical and histopathological prognostic factors
  - Here, prognostic factors for groin LN metastases on the basis of the entire data set (findings on superficial lesions published earlier); since histologic groin node status the most important independent prognostic factor for death
- **Results:**
  - 637 enrolled and 588 evaluable
  - 18.9% with LN metastases for tumors ≤2 cm
  - 41.6% for tumors >2 cm
  - 23.9% of 477 patients with clinically unsuspicious nodes had surgically positive LNs
    - Body weight not related to sensitivity of detecting positive LNs clinically (p = 0.26)
  - Independent risk factors for positive LNs identified (in order of importance)
    - Less tumor differentiation by GOG criteria (p < 0.0001)
    - Suspicious or fixed/ulcerated LNs (p < 0.0001)
    - Capillary-lymphatic involvement (p < 0.0001)
    - Older age (p = 0.0002)
    - Greater tumor thickness (invasion) (p = 0.03)
      - ≤1 mm: 2.6% with positive groin LN
  - Lesion size and location were not independent predictors of positive LNs

Study: GOG 74

- **Citation:** (Stehman et al., 1992a)
- **Highlight:** Radical hemivulvectomy with ipsilateral superficial LND

- **Design:**
  - From 1983 to 1989, 155 patients with clinical stage I enrolled in a prospective study evaluating modified radical hemivulvectomy and ipsilateral superficial inguinal lymphadenectomy (cribriform fascia left intact)
    - Eligible only
      - Neoplastic thickness: ≤5 mm
      - No LVSI
      - Negative inguinal LNs
- **Results:**
  - 19/121 evaluated patients recurred
    - 8/10 local vulvar recurrences salvaged by further surgery
  - 7/121 died from disease
    - 5/7 first recurred in groin
  - Acute and long-term morbidity and hospital stay less than in population treated with radical vulvectomy and bilateral IFL
  - Increased risk of recurrence but not death when compared with historic control
- **Conclusion:**
  - → Modified radical hemivulvectomy and ipsilateral inguinal lymphadenectomy is alternative to traditional radical operation for stage I vulva cancer
  - Number of groin recurrences may be attributable to decision to leave femoral LNs intact

Study: Te Grootenhuis study

- **Citation:** (Te Grootenhuis et al., 2019)
- **Highlight:** Local recurrence in relation to tumor- and precursor lesion-free margins
- **Design:**
  - 287 patients with surgically treated primary vulvar squamous cell carcinoma included
- **Results:**
  - Median follow-up: 80 months
  - 10-yr actuarial local recurrence rate: 42.5%
  - Margin distance did not influence local recurrence, neither using cutoff of 8, 5, and 3 mm (HR 1.03 [CI = 0.99–1.06])
  - Multivariable analyses showed higher local recurrence with dVIN and lichen sclerosus in the margin (HR 2.76 [CI = 1.62–4.71]), stage II or higher (HR 1.62 [CI = 1.05–2.48])
- **Conclusion:**
  - → Local recurrences are frequent and are associated with dVIN (with or without lichen sclerosus) in the margin rather than any tumor-free margin distance

4.1.1 Groin Lymph Nodes

Study: GOG 88

- **Citation:** (Stehman et al., 1992b)
- **Highlight:** Groin irradiation vs. LND for clinically negative LNs
- **Design:**
  - To determine if groin radiation superior to groin dissection and less morbid
  - 58 patients with primary stage I–III (stage I only eligible if positive LVSI or >5 mm invasion) squamous cell carcinoma of vulva and non-suspicious inguinal nodes (N0–1) randomized to radical vulvectomy + groin dissection vs. radical vulvectomy + groin radiation
  - Radiation: 50 Gy in daily 2 Gy fractions to depth of 3 cm below anterior skin surface
- **Results:**
  - Study closed prematurely when interim analysis revealed excessive number of groin relapses on groin radiation regimen
  - LN involvement predicted in 24% (based on GOG 36)
  - In groin dissection group, 5/25 (20%) found to have positive LNs; these patients received postoperative radiation
  - 5/27 (18.5%) groin relapses in radiation group and none in groin dissection group
  - Statistically significant difference in PSF ($p = 0.03$) and survival ($p = 0.04$)
- **Conclusion:**
  - → Radiation to intact groins significantly inferior to groin dissection in squamous cell carcinoma of vulva and N0–1 nodes

Study: GROINSS-V-I (GROningen INternational Study on Sentinel Nodes in Vulvar Cancer)

- **Citation:** (Van der Zee et al., 2008)
- **Highlight:** SLN sampling in early-stage vulvar cancer
- **Design:**
  - March 2000 to June 2006: Multicenter observational study on SLN detection using radioactive tracer and blue dye in T1 and T2 (<4 cm) squamous cell carcinoma of vulva in 623 groins of 403 patients
  - When SLN negative on ultrastaging, IFL omitted and patient observed with follow-up for 2 yrs q 2 months
- **Results:**
  - In 259 patients with unifocal disease, negative SLNs and median follow-up of 35 months, six groin recurrences (2.3%) and 3-yr survival 97%
  - Short-term morbidity (SLN sampling vs. IFL)
    - Wound breakdown groin: 11.7% vs. 34% ($p < 0.0001$)
    - Cellulitis: 4.5% vs. 21.3% ($p < 0.0001$)

- Long-term morbidity
  - Recurrent erysipelas: 0.4% vs. 16.2% (p < 0.0001)
  - Lymphedema: 1.9% vs. 25.2% (p < 0.0001)
- **Conclusion:**
  - → In early-stage vulvar cancer with negative SLN, groin recurrence rate low, survival excellent, and treatment-related morbidity minimal

Study: GROINSS-V-I

- **Citation:** (Oonk et al., 2010)
- **Highlight:** Size of SLN metastasis and chance of non-SLN involvement
- **Design:**
  - Metastatic disease in one or more SLNs in 135 (33%) of 403 patients
    - 115/135 (85%) underwent IFL
  - Risk of non-sentinel-node metastasis higher when positive SLN found on routine pathology vs. ultrastaging (23/85 vs. 3/56 groins; p = 0.001)
  - 723 SLNs in 260 patients reviewed (i.e., 2.8 SLN per patient)
  - Proportion of patients with non-SLN metastasis increased with size of SLN metastasis
    - 1/24 patients with individual tumor cells with non-SLN metastasis
    - 2/19 with micro-metastasis (≤2 mm)
    - 2/15 with metastasis >2 to 5 mm
    - 10/21 with metastasis >5 mm
  - Disease-specific survival for patients with SLN metastasis >2 mm lower than for those with micro-metastasis (≤2 mm): 69.5% vs. 94.4% (p = 0.001)
- **Conclusion:**
  - → Risk of non-SLN metastasis increases with size of SLN metastasis; no size cutoff seems to exist below which chance of non-SLN close to zero
  - All patients with SLN metastasis should have additional groin treatment

Study: GROINSS-V-I

- **Citation:** (Te Grootenhuis et al., 2016)
- **Highlight:** Long-term follow-up
- **Results:**
  - Median follow-up: 105 months
  - Overall local 5-yr and 10-yr recurrence rate: 27.2% and 39.5%
    - For SLN-negative patients: 24.6% and 36.4%
    - For SLN-positive patients: 33.2% and 46.4% (p = 0.03)
  - In 39/253 (15.4%) SLN-negative patients: IFL performed because of local recurrence
  - Isolated 5-yr groin recurrence
    - In SLN-negative patients: 2.5%
    - In SLN-positive patients: 8%

- 10-yr disease-specific survival: 91% vs. 65% (SLN-negative vs. SLN-positive) (p = 0.0001)
- For all patients, 10-yr disease-specific survival decreased from 90% to 69% with local recurrence (p = 0.001)

Study: GOG 173

- **Citation:** (Levenback et al., 2012)
- **Highlight:** Evaluation of SLN sampling with complete LND in early-stage vulvar cancer
- **Design:**
  - To determine safety of SLN to replace inguinal femoral lymphadenectomy
  - From 1999 to 2009, 452 patients with squamous cell carcinoma of vulva, at least 1 mm invasion, tumor size ≥2 and ≤6 cm, limited to vulva and clinically negative LNs underwent lymphatic mapping, SLN biopsy, and inguinal femoral lymphadenectomy
  - Ultrastaging of the SLN
  - Intradermal injection of isosulfan blue and radioactive tracer; intraoperative gamma counter: 10× of background
  - Initially, preoperative scintigraphy optional; 2 yrs into the study (required)
- **Results:**
  - In 418/452, at least one SLN identified
  - 132 node-positive
  - 11/132 (8.3%) false-negative
  - IHC performed on 200/285 patients with negative SLN on H&E; 23% (28 patients) detected by IHC alone (in 55% SLN was the only positive LN; not indicated what percentage was detected by IHC alone)
  - Sensitivity: 91.7%; false-negative rate (1-sensitivity) = 8.3%
  - False-negative predictive value (1–negative predictive value) = 3.7%
  - In women with less than 4 cm tumors, false-negative predictive value = 2.0%
- **Conclusion:**
  - → SLN biopsy reasonable alternative to inguinal femoral lymphadenectomy in selected women with squamous cell carcinoma of vulva

Study: GROINSS-V-II

- **Citation:** (Oonk et al., 2021)
- **Background:**
  - To investigate safety of omitting IFL in SLN-positive patients and replacing it with adjuvant radiotherapy; inguinofemoral radiotherapy could spare vulvar cancer patients with SLN micrometastases the morbidity of lymphadenectomy
- **Design:**
  - In phase II single-arm treatment trial, 322 patients with early-stage vulvar cancer (diameter <4 cm) without signs of LN involvement on imaging;

SLN biopsy was performed; when SLN involved with metastasis of any size, inguinofemoral radiotherapy was given (50 Gy)

- **Results:**
  - After 91 SLN-positive patients included, stopping rule activated because of high groin recurrence; 9/10 patients with groin recurrence showed SLN metastasis of >2 mm and/or extracapsular spread
  - Protocol amended: Those with SLN macrometastases (>2 mm) underwent IFL; those with micrometastases (≤2 mm) received inguinofemoral radiotherapy
  - 126/160 patients with SLN micrometastasis received inguinofemoral radiation
    - Ipsilateral groin recurrence rate at 2 yrs of 1.6%
  - 51/162 with SLN macrometastases received inguinofemoral radiation
    - Ipsilateral groin recurrence rate at 2 yrs of 22%
  - 105/162 with SLN macrometastases underwent IFL
    - 59/105 received additional radiation
    - Ipsilateral groin recurrence rate (IFL with or without RT) at 2 yrs of 6.9%
- **Conclusion:**
  - → Inguinofemoral radiation is a safe alternative to IFL in patients with SLN micrometastases with minimal morbidity. For patients with SLN macrometastases, RT with total of 50 Gy resulted in more groin recurrences compared with IFL

4.2 STUDIES ADDRESSING ADVANCED VULVAR CANCER

4.2.1 Chemoradiation

Study: GOG 101

- **Citation:** (Moore et al., 1998)
- **Highlight:** Preoperative chemoRT in advanced-stage vulvar cancer
- **Design:**
  - To determine feasibility of preoperative chemoRT to avert need for more radical surgery for T3 tumors or pelvic exenteration for T4 tumors
  - Phase II study: 73 patients with clinical stage III–IV squamous cell carcinoma of vulva received concurrent cisplatin (50 mg/m^2) and 5-fluorouracil (1,000 mg/m^2/d × 4 d) q 4 wks, and RT followed by radical surgical excision of residual tumor + bilateral inguinofemoral LND

- Split-course chemoRT: With CT twice-daily RT (days 1–4) to primary tumor by AP-PA fields, then daily RT (days 5–12); then treatment break; then on day 29 CT with twice-daily RT (days 29–32), then daily RT (days 33–40) (total 28 fractions of 1.7 Gy; total 47.6 Gy); patients with inoperable groin LNs received chemoRT to primary vulva tumor, inguinofemoral, and lower PLNs
- **Results:**
  - For seven patients, no post-treatment surgical procedure
  - 33/71 (46.5%) had no visible disease
  - 38/71 (53.5%) with gross residual
  - 5/38 with positive margins
    - 3/5 further RT to vulva
    - 1/5 wide local excision and vaginectomy necessitating colostomy
    - 1/5 NFT
  - Only 2/71 (2.8%) with residual unresectable disease
  - Only 3/71: Not possible to preserve urinary and/or GI continence
  - Toxicity acceptable
    - Cutaneous reactions to chemoRT and surgical wound complications most common AEs
- **Conclusion:**
  - → Preoperative chemoRT in advanced squamous cell carcinoma of vulva feasible and may reduce need for more radical surgery

Study: GOG 205

- **Citation:** (Moore et al., 2012)
- **Highlight:** ChemoRT in advanced vulva cancer
- **Design:**
  - Phase II trial to determine efficacy and toxicity of chemoRT as primary treatment of locally advanced vulvar cancer
  - 58 patients with primary locally advanced (T2 and T4 tumors amenable to radical vulvectomy) treated with 1.8 Gy qd × 32 fractions (57.6 Gy) + cisplatin 40 mg/m^2 q wk followed by surgical resection of residual tumor (or biopsy to confirm complete clinical response)
  - Primary endpoint: Complete clinical and pathological response of the primary vulvar cancer
  - Management of groin LN
    - If clinically negative or resectable, pretreatment inguinal–femoral LND
      - If pathology negative, decision whether or not RT to groin up to the discretion of treating physician
- **Results:**
  - 40/58 patients (69%) completed the study
  - Discontinuation of treatment for
    - Refusal (four), toxicity (nine), death (two), and other (three)
  - Clinical CR: 37/58 (64%)

- 34 underwent biopsy → 29/34 (78%) also with complete pathological response
- AEs
  - Leukopenia
  - Pain
  - Radiation dermatitis
  - Metabolic changes
- **Conclusion:**
  - → Combination of RT and weekly cisplatin yielded high clinical and pathological response rates with acceptable toxicity
  - Comparison to GOG 101
    - Cisplatin only (no 5-FU) with RT
    - No planned treatment break
    - 20% increased RT dose

4.2.2 Immunotherapy

Study: Keynote-158

- **Citation:** (Shapira-Frommer et al., 2022)
- **Highlight:** Pembrolizumab in advanced vulva cancer
- **Design:**
  - Phase II multicohort trial: 101 patients with advanced vulvar squamous cell carcinoma received 200 mg pembrolizumab iv q 3 wks for up to 35 C
  - Subgroup: PD-L1-positive (CPS ≥1) and PD-L1-negative (CPS <1)
- **Results:**
  - ORR: 10.9%
    - 9.5% among 84 PD-L1-positive tumors
    - 28.6% among seven PD-L1-negative tumors
    - Median DOR: 20.4 months
  - Median PFS: 2.1 months
  - Median OS: 6.2 months
  - ≥ Grade 3 AEs in 11.9%
- **Conclusion:**
  - → Pembrolizumab associated with durable response in a subset of vulvar SCC, regardless of PD-L1 status

REFERENCES

Homesley, H.D., Bundy, B.N., Sedlis, A., Yordan, E., Berek, J.S., Jahshan, A., and Mortel, R. (1993). Prognostic factors for groin node metastasis in squamous cell carcinoma of the vulva (a Gynecologic Oncology Group study). Gynecol Oncol 49, 279–283. 10.1006/gyno.1993.1127.

Levenback, C.F., Ali, S., Coleman, R.L., Gold, M.A., Fowler, J.M., Judson, P.L., Bell, M.C., De Geest, K., Spirtos, N.M., Potkul, R.K., et al. (2012). Lymphatic mapping and sentinel lymph node biopsy in women with squamous cell carcinoma of the vulva: a Gynecologic Oncology Group study. J Clin Oncol *30*, 3786–3791. 10.1200/JCO.2011.41.2528.

Moore, D.H., Ali, S., Koh, W.J., Michael, H., Barnes, M.N., McCourt, C.K., Homesley, H.D., and Walker, J.L. (2012). A phase II trial of radiation therapy and weekly cisplatin chemotherapy for the treatment of locally-advanced squamous cell carcinoma of the vulva: a Gynecologic Oncology Group study. Gynecol Oncol *124*, 529–533. 10.1016/j.ygyno.2011.11.003.

Moore, D.H., Thomas, G.M., Montana, G.S., Saxer, A., Gallup, D.G., and Olt, G. (1998). Preoperative chemoradiation for advanced vulvar cancer: a phase II study of the Gynecologic Oncology Group. Int J Radiat Oncol Biol Phys *42*, 79–85.

Oonk, M.H.M., Slomovitz, B., Baldwin, P.J.W., Doorn, H.C.v., Velden, J.v.d., Hullu, J.A.d., Gaarenstroom, K.N., Slangen, B.F.M., Vergote, I., Brännström, M., et al. (2021). Radiotherapy versus inguinofemoral lymphadenectomy as treatment for vulvar cancer patients with micrometastases in the sentinel node: results of GROINSS-V II. J Clin Oncol *39*, 3623–3632. 10.1200/jco.21.00006.

Oonk, M.H., van Hemel, B.M., Hollema, H., de Hullu, J.A., Ansink, A.C., Vergote, I., Verheijen, R.H., Maggioni, A., Gaarenstroom, K.N., Baldwin, P.J., et al. (2010). Size of sentinel-node metastasis and chances of non-sentinel-node involvement and survival in early stage vulvar cancer: results from GROINSS-V, a multicentre observational study. Lancet Oncol *11*, 646–652. 10.1016/S1470-2045(10)70104-2.

Sedlis, A., Homesley, H., Bundy, B.N., Marshall, R., Yordan, E., Hacker, N., Lee, J.H., and Whitney, C. (1987). Positive groin lymph nodes in superficial squamous cell vulvar cancer. a Gynecologic Oncology Group study. Am J Obstet Gynecol *156*, 1159–1164.

Shapira-Frommer, R., Mileshkin, L., Manzyuk, L., Penel, N., Burge, M., Piha-Paul, S.A., Girda, E., Lopez Martin, J.A., van Dongen, M.G.J., Italiano, A., et al. (2022). Efficacy and safety of pembrolizumab for patients with previously treated advanced vulvar squamous cell carcinoma: results from the phase 2 KEYNOTE-158 study. Gynecol Oncol. 10.1016/j.ygyno.2022.01.029.

Stehman, F.B., Bundy, B.N., Dvoretsky, P.M., and Creasman, W.T. (1992a). Early stage I carcinoma of the vulva treated with ipsilateral superficial inguinal lymphadenectomy and modified radical hemivulvectomy: a prospective study of the Gynecologic Oncology Group. Obstet Gynecol *79*, 490–497.

Stehman, F.B., Bundy, B.N., Thomas, G., Varia, M., Okagaki, T., Roberts, J., Bell, J., and Heller, P.B. (1992b). Groin dissection versus groin radiation in carcinoma of the vulva: a Gynecologic Oncology Group study. Int J Radiat Oncol Biol Phys *24*, 389–396.

Te Grootenhuis, N.C., Pouwer, A.W., de Bock, G.H., Hollema, H., Bulten, J., van der Zee, A.G.J., de Hullu, J.A., and Oonk, M.H.M. (2019). Margin status revisited in vulvar squamous cell carcinoma. Gynecol Oncol *154*, 266–275. 10.1016/j.ygyno.2019.05.010.

Te Grootenhuis, N.C., van der Zee, A.G., van Doorn, H.C., van der Velden, J., Vergote, I., Zanagnolo, V., Baldwin, P.J., Gaarenstroom, K.N., van Dorst, E.B., Trum, J.W., et al. (2016). Sentinel nodes in vulvar cancer: long-term follow-up of the GROningen INternational study on Sentinel nodes in vulvar cancer (GROINSS-V) I. Gynecol Oncol *140*, 8–14. 10.1016/j.ygyno.2015.09.077.

Van der Zee, A.G., Oonk, M.H., De Hullu, J.A., Ansink, A.C., Vergote, I., Verheijen, R.H., Maggioni, A., Gaarenstroom, K.N., Baldwin, P.J., Van Dorst, E.B., et al. (2008). Sentinel node dissection is safe in the treatment of early-stage vulvar cancer. J Clin Oncol *26*, 884–889. 10.1200/JCO.2007.14.0566.

Gestational Trophoblastic Neoplasia

5

5.1 STUDIES ADDRESSING SURGICAL TREATMENT

Study: GOG 242

- **Citation:** (Osborne et al., 2016)
- **Highlight:** Second curettage for low-risk non-metastatic gestational trophoblastic neoplasia (GTN)
- **Design:**
  - Phase II: 60 patients with newly diagnosed low-risk (defined as WHO risk score 0–6) non-metastatic GTN received second uterine curettage
- **Results:**
  - 24 patients (40%) cured
  - CR: Additional two patients but lost to follow-up
  - 26/60 (43%) able to avoid CT
  - 34/60 (59%) surgical failure
    - More common in age ≤19 or ≤40
    - In three cases: Placental site trophoblastic tumor
    - In one case: Placental nodule
  - AEs
    - Uterine perforation grade 1: 1
    - Uterine hemorrhage grade 1: 4; grade 3: 1
- **Conclusion:**
  - Second uterine curettage as initial treatment for low-risk non-metastatic GTN cures 40%; no significant morbidity

Study: Eysbouts study

- **Citation:** (Eysbouts et al., 2017)
- **Highlight:** Hysterectomy for GTN

DOI: 10.1201/9781003229711-5

- **Design:**
  - Retrospective study of 109 patients from Dutch national database with GTN who underwent hysterectomy
- **Results:**
  - 74.3% with low-risk GTN; 73.5% post-molar GTN; 65.1% confined to uterus
  - After hysterectomy
    - CR: 66.2% in patients with localized disease
    - CR: 15.8% in patients with metastatic disease
    - Localized disease treated with primary hysterectomy
      - Treatment duration: 3.2 vs. 8.0 wks (p = 0.01) (with vs. without)
      - CT cycles: 1.5 vs. 5.8 (p < 0.01)
- **Conclusion:**
  - → In select cases, hysterectomy may be effective to reduce or eliminate tumor bulk
  - Primary hysterectomy may be considered in older patients with localized disease and completed childbearing.
  - Patients with CT-resistant disease may benefit from additional hysterectomy
    - Especially when disease localized
    - Removal of tumor bulk in widespread disease

5.2 STUDIES ADDRESSING CHEMOTHERAPY IN LOW-RISK GESTATIONAL TROPHOBLASTIC NEOPLASIA

Study: GOG 174

- **Citation:** (Osborne et al., 2011)
- **Highlight:** Dactinomycin vs. weekly MTX in low-risk GTN
- **Design:**
  - 216 patients with low-risk GTN randomized to dactinomycin 1.25 mg/m^2 q 2 wks vs. MTX IM 30 mg/m^2 q wk
  - Patients with WHO score 0–6; metastatic disease (limited to lung lesions <2 cm, adnexa, or vagina); non-metastatic choriocarcinoma
- **Results:**
  - CR: 70% vs. 53% (p = 0.01) (dactinomycin vs. MTX)
    - Low risk (WHO risk score 0–4 and excluding choriocarcinoma)
      - CR: 73% vs. 58% (p = 0.03)
    - WHO risk score 5–6 or choriocarcinoma
      - CR: 42% vs. 7%
  - Both regimens well tolerated
- **Conclusion:**
  - → Biweekly dactinomycin with higher CR than weekly MTX in low-risk GTN

Study: Cochrane review

- **Citation:** (Lawrie et al., 2016)
- **Highlight:** First-line CT in low-risk GTN
- **Design:**
  - Meta-analysis of RCTs, quasi-RCTs, and non-RCTs
- **Results:**
  - Six RCTs (667 women) included
  - Three studies compared weekly IM MTX with bi-weekly pulsed iv actinomycin; one study 5-d IM MTX with bi-weekly pulsed iv actinomycin; one study 8-d IM MTX–folinic acid with 5-d iv actinomycin; one study 8-d MTX–folinic acid with bi-weekly pulsed iv actinomycin
  - Moderate-certainty evidence
    - Actinomycin D more likely to lead to primary cure than MTX (RR 0.65 [CI = 0.57–0.75])
    - MTX more likely to fail than actinomycin D (RR 3.55 [CI: +1.81–6.95])
  - Low-certainty evidence
    - No difference in nausea: RR 0.61 (CI = 0.29–1.26)
    - Little or no difference in risk of sAEs (RR 0.35 [CI = 0.08–1.66]); however, direction favors MTX
  - No evidence on effect on future fertility
- **Conclusion:**
  - → Pulsed actinomycin D is more likely to achieve primary cure in low-risk GTN and less likely treatment failure than MTX
  - High-certainty data are still needed

Study: GOG 275

- **Citation:** (Schink et al., 2020)
- **Highlight:** Actinomycin D vs. multiday MTX
- **Design:**
  - In non-inferior trial, 54 patients with low-risk GTN randomized to pulsed 1.25 mg/m^2 actinomycin D iv q 2 wks vs. multiday 50 mg MTX IM on days 1, 3, 5, and 7 with 15 mg folinic acid rescue po on days 2, 4, 6, and 8 or single-agent MTX 0.4 mg/kg iv (25 mg maximum daily dose) on days 1–5 q 2 wks
  - Continue study treatment for 3 C after hCG <5 mIU/mL, disease progression, or toxicity
  - Study was closed for low accrual
- **Results:**
  - CR: 88% (23/26) multiday MTX
  - CR: 79% (22/28) actinomycin D
  - Two recurrences in each arm
  - Mucositis (p = 0.001) and eye pain (p = 0.01) more common in MTX arm
- **Conclusion:**
  - → CR higher for multiday MTX but did not reach statistical significance; multiday MTX with more mucositis and less convenient

5.3 STUDIES ADDRESSING (CHEMO)THERAPY IN HIGH-RISK GESTATIONAL TROPHOBLASTIC NEOPLASIA

Study: Alifrangis EMA/CO study

- **Citation:** (Alifrangis et al., 2013)
- **Highlight:** EMA/CO for high-risk GTN
- **Background:**
  - For high-risk GTN, frequently etoposide, MTX, dactinomycin alternating with cyclophosphamide and vincristine
  - 1979–1995: OS 85.4% with significant portion of early deaths
- **Design:**
  - Retrospective study of 438 patients who received EMA/CO between 1995 and 2010
  - Genetic analyses identified non-gestational trophoblastic tumors (nGTTs)
  - EMA/CO
    - Day 1: Etoposide 100 mg/m^2 for 30 min, dactinomycin 0.5 mg iv bolus, and MTX 300 mg/m^2 for 12 hrs
    - Day 2: Etoposide 100 mg/m^2 for 30 min, dactinomycin 0.5 mg iv bolus, and folinic acid rescue 15 mg iv or orally every 12 hrs × 4 doses commencing 24 hrs after starting MTX
    - Day 8: Vincristine 1 mg/m^2 iv bolus and cyclophosphamide 600 mg/m^2 iv for 30 min
    - 14-day cycle (EMA alternates with CO every week)
  - Use of induction low-dose etoposide 100 mg/m^2 and cisplatin 20 mg/m^2 on days 1 and 2 q wk × 1–2 C in select patients at high risk for early death (i.e., with extensive disease in chest, liver, brain, FIGO score >12, and/or major bleeding)
- **Results:**
  - 6/438 patients with nGTTs
  - 140/438 patients with high-risk disease
  - 250/438 patients with relapsed/resistant low-risk GTN
  - Median follow-up time: 4.2 yrs
  - OS in high-risk patients: 94.3% (90.4% including nGTTs)
  - OS in low-risk patients: 99.6%
  - 6/6 patients with nGTTs and seven patients with high-risk GTN died of drug-resistant disease
  - EP induction CT in 33/140 (23.1%) high-risk patients with larger disease burden
    - Early death rate only 0.7% vs. 7.2% in the pre-1995 cohort

- **Conclusion:**
  - → OS for high-risk GTN increased by nearly 9%
    - More accurate by excluding nGTTs (3/9%) with genetic analysis
    - Low-dose induction EP allows near-complete resolution of early deaths

Study: Ghorani pembrolizumab study

- **Citation:** (Ghorani et al., 2017)
- **Highlight:** Pembrolizumab in GTN
- **Background:**
  - Placental expression of paternal antigens makes placenta target for maternal immune recognition; PD-L1 expression maintains gestational tolerance
  - PD-L1 strongly expressed by GTN
- **Design:** Four cases reported
- **Results:**
  - 39 yo with high-risk choriocarcinoma progressed through fifth line, with 100% PD-L1 expression, and rich in TILs normalized serum hCG after four cycles of pembrolizumab and after four additional cycles remain in complete remission over 24 months
  - 44 yo with PSTT/ETT s/p multiple failed lines, >90% PD-L1 positive but negative for TILs progressed after five cycles of pembrolizumab and died 4 months later
  - 47 yo with metastatic PSTT progressing through third-line treatment, >90% PD-L1 positive and presence of TILs; after eight cycles of pembrolizumab serum hCG normalized, plus five consolidation cycles patient remains in remission over 15 months
  - 37 yo with lung metastatic choriocarcinoma in remission after five lines of CT, with 100% PD-L1 expression, and dense TILs; on relapse received pembrolizumab; after two cycles remission and remains in remission after four additional cycles over 5 months
  - In all cases only grade 1–2 AEs
- **Conclusion:**
  - → For unresectable drug resistant GTNs anti-PD1 immunotherapy may be effective
  - Caveat lasting fertility impairment (persistent anti-trophoblastic immunity)
  - PD-L1, TILs, and HL-G may be important identifiers of responders

Study: TROPHIMMUN—Cohort A

- **Citation:** (You et al., 2020)
- **Highlight:** Avelumab in GTN resistant to single-agent CT
- **Background:**
  - Standard treatment for GTN resistant to CT includes single agent or polychemotherapy, is effective (65–95% hCG normalization) and toxic; PD-L1 constitutively expressed in all GTN subtypes

- **Design:**
  - Phase II two-cohort trial; cohort A: GTN resistant to monochemotherapy; cohort B: GTN resistant to polychemotherapy; here, results of cohort A reported.
  - 10 mg/kg avelumab iv q 2 wks until hCG normalization, followed by three consolidation cycles
- **Results:**
  - 15 patients treated
  - Median age: 34
  - Stage I: 53.3%; stage III: 46.7%
  - FIGO score: 0–4 in 33.3%, 5–6 in 46.7%, and ≥7 in 20%
  - Prior treatment: MTX (100%) and actinomycin D (7%)
  - Median follow-up: 25 months
  - 53.3% with hCG normalization after median of 9 C avelumab; none relapsed
  - Probability of hCG normalization not associated with stage, FIGO score, or baseline hCG
  - One patient with subsequent healthy pregnancy
  - 46.7% avelumab resistant: hCG normalized with actinomycin D in 42.3% or combination CT/surgery (57.1%)
  - Grade 1–2 AEs: 33.3% fatigue, 33.3% nausea/vomiting, and 26.7% infusion-related reaction
- **Conclusion:**
  - → In patients with single-agent CT-resistant GTN avelumab with favorable safety profile and cured 50% of patients; avelumab could be new therapeutic option, particularly if otherwise combination CT required

Study: TROPHIMMUN—Cohort B

- **Citation:** NCT03135769, presented at ESGO 2021, ongoing, (You et al., 2021)
- **Highlight:** Avelumab in GTN resistant to polychemotherapy
- **Background:**
  - GTN with FIGO score ≥7, resistant to both standard monotherapies; EMA-CO is recommended; if resistant to polychemotherapy, prognosis is poor.
- **Results:**
  - Cohort B closed for futility
  - Seven patients treated
  - Stage I: 43%; stage III: 57%
  - FIGO score: 8–10 in 43%; 11–15 in 57%
  - Six patients achieved initial hCG stabilization/decline
  - One patient with hCG normalization after 13 cycles; another patient with hCG decline, and then underwent hemostatic hysterectomy, five (You et al., 2021), five other patients experienced hCG re-increase

- **Conclusion:**
  - → Contrarily to cohort A, avelumab activity was limited in patients with polychemotherapy resistance; hCG normalization was rare (14%); prognosis of patients experiencing polychemotherapy remains poor

Study: CAP 01

- **Citation:** (Cheng et al., 2021)
- **Highlight:** Camrelizumab plus apatinib in high-risk chemorefractory or relapsed GTN
- **Design:**
  - Single-arm phase II trial: 20 patients with high-risk (FIGO score ≥7) chemorefractory or relapsed GTN with ≥2 prior lines of multidrug CT received 200 mg camrelizumab iv q 2 wks plus 250 mg apatinib po qd
  - Camrelizumab is a PD-1 antibody. Apatinib is a tyrosine kinase inhibitor selectively binding to VEGFR2
- **Results:**
  - 19 with choriocarcinoma; one with placental site trophoblastic tumor
  - Median follow-up: 18.5 months
  - ORR: 55%
    - CR: 50% (10/20)
  - ≥ Grade 3 AEs: Hypertension (25%), neutropenia (10%), leukopenia (10%), and AST elevation (10%)
- **Conclusion:**
  - → Camrelizumab plus apatinib with promising antitumor activity and acceptable toxicity could be salvage therapy option in high-risk chemorefractory or relapsed GTN

REFERENCES

Alifrangis, C., Agarwal, R., Short, D., Fisher, R.A., Sebire, N.J., Harvey, R., Savage, P.M., and Seckl, M.J. (2013). EMA/CO for high-risk gestational trophoblastic neoplasia: good outcomes with induction low-dose etoposide-cisplatin and genetic analysis. J Clin Oncol *31*, 280–286. 10.1200/JCO.2012.43.1817.

Cheng, H., Zong, L., Kong, Y., Wang, X., Gu, Y., Cang, W., Zhao, J., Wan, X., Yang, J., and Xiang, Y. (2021). Camrelizumab plus apatinib in patients with high-risk chemorefractory or relapsed gestational trophoblastic neoplasia (CAP 01): a single-arm, open-label, phase 2 trial. Lancet Oncol *22*, 1609–1617. 10.1016/S1470-2045(21)00460-5.

Eysbouts, Y.K., Massuger, L., IntHout, J., Lok, C.A.R., Sweep, F., and Ottevanger, P.B. (2017). The added value of hysterectomy in the management of gestational trophoblastic neoplasia. Gynecol Oncol *145*, 536–542. 10.1016/j.ygyno.2017.03.018.

Ghorani, E., Kaur, B., Fisher, R.A., Short, D., Joneborg, U., Carlson, J.W., Akarca, A., Marafioti, T., Quezada, S.A., Sarwar, N., and Seckl, M.J. (2017). Pembrolizumab is effective for drug-resistant gestational trophoblastic neoplasia. Lancet *390*, 2343–2345. 10.1016/S0140–6736(17)32894-5.

Lawrie, T.A., Alazzam, M., Tidy, J., Hancock, B.W., and Osborne, R. (2016). First-line chemotherapy in low-risk gestational trophoblastic neoplasia. Cochrane Database Syst Rev, CD007102. 10.1002/14651858.CD007102.pub4.

Osborne, R.J., Filiaci, V.L., Schink, J.C., Mannel, R.S., Alvarez Secord, A., Kelley, J.L., Provencher, D., Scott Miller, D., Covens, A.L., and Lage, J.M. (2011). Phase III trial of weekly methotrexate or pulsed dactinomycin for low-risk gestational trophoblastic neoplasia: a Gynecologic Oncology Group study. J Clin Oncol 29, 825–831. 10.1200/JCO.2010.30.4386.

Osborne, R.J., Filiaci, V.L., Schink, J.C., Mannel, R.S., Behbakht, K., Hoffman, J.S., Spirtos, N.M., Chan, J.K., Tidy, J.A., and Miller, D.S. (2016). Second curettage for low-risk nonmetastatic gestational trophoblastic neoplasia. Obstet Gynecol 128, 535–542. 10.1097/AOG.0000000000001554.

Schink, J.C., Filiaci, V., Huang, H.Q., Tidy, J., Winter, M., Carter, J., Anderson, N., Moxley, K., Yabuno, A., Taylor, S.E., et al. (2020). An international randomized phase III trial of pulse actinomycin-D versus multi-day methotrexate for the treatment of low risk gestational trophoblastic neoplasia; NRG/GOG 275. Gynecol Oncol 158, 354–360. 10.1016/j.ygyno.2020.05.013.

You, B., Bolze, P.-A, Lotz, J., Massardier, J., Gladieff, L., Floquet, A., Hajri, T., Descargues, P., Langlois-Jacques, C., Mercier, C., et al. (2021). 273 Avelumab in patients with gestational trophoblastic tumorsresistant to polychemotherapy: efficacy outcomes of cohort B of TROPHIMMUN phase II trial. Int J Gynecol Cancer 31, A344–A344. 10.1136/ijgc-2021-ESGO.608.

You, B., Bolze, P.-A., Lotz, J.-P., Massardier, J., Gladieff, L., Joly, F., Hajri, T., Maucort-Boulch, D., Bin, S., Rousset, P., et al. (2020). Avelumab in patients with gestational trophoblastic tumors with resistance to single-agent chemotherapy: cohort A of the TROPHIMMUN phase II trial. J Clin Oncol 38, 3129–3137. 10.1200/jco.20.00803.

Glossary

AE	adverse event
AGO	Arbeitsgruppe Onkologie
AUC	area under the curve
BID	*bis in die* [twice a day]
C	cycle
CBR	clinical benefit rate
CI	confidence interval
CR	complete response
CT	chemotherapy
CTRT	chemo-radiation therapy
d	day
DFI	disease-free interval
EBRT	external beam radiation therapy
FFS	failure-free survival
FIGO	International Federation of Gynecology and Obstetrics
GOG	Gynecologic Oncology Group
HR	hazard ratio
ICBT	intracavitary brachytherapy
IFL	inguinofemoral lymphadenectomy
IHC	immunohistochemistry
IMRT	intensity-modulated radiation therapy
LOH	loss of heterozygosity
LVSI	lymphovascular space invasion
NACT	neoadjuvant chemotherapy
NFT	no further treatment
NPV	negative predictive value
OR	operating room
ORR	objective response rate
OS	overall survival
PD	progressive disease
PFS	progression-free survival
PLND	pelvic lymph node dissection
PR	partial response
q	every
RCT	randomized control trial
RFS	recurrence-free survival
RT	radiation therapy
RTOG	Radiation Therapy Oncology Group
SD	stable disease

SLN	sentinel lymph node
vs.	versus
wk	week
yr	year

Index

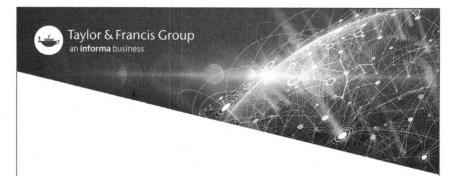

Printed in the United States
by Baker & Taylor Publisher Services